LOST & FOUND

A Survivor's Guide for Reconstructing Life After a Brain Injury

Lighting the Way with Tips, Tools and Strategies

By Barbara J. Webster

ISBN 978-1-931117-61-6

Item: LFSG

Published by Lash & Associates Publishing/Training Inc.
100 Boardwalk Drive, Suite 150, Youngsville, NC 27596
Tel: (919) 556-0300

This book is part of a series on brain injury among children, adolescents, adults and veterans.
For a free catalog, contact Lash & Associates
Tel: (919) 556-0300 or visit our web site *www.lapublishing.com*

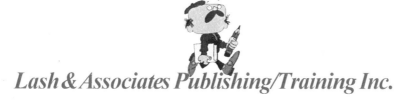

Lash & Associates Publishing/Training Inc.

Dedication

This guide is dedicated to The "Amazing" Brain Injury Survivor Support Group in Framingham, MA. and brain injury survivors everywhere who are bravely striving to thrive while struggling with cognitive difficulties. Their never-ending courage and determination to be all that they can be is inspiring and truly amazing. Without their caring and sharing, this book would not have happened!

"We are human "beings", not human "thinkings."

— Deepak Chopra

Acknowledgements

With much gratitude I want to thank all of the truly exceptional people who work and live with brain injury survivors, both professionals and non-professionals. It has been my good fortune to know and learn from many of them. One of the greatest gifts a survivor can have is the support of family and friends. They provide the foundation for healing. I truly might not be here today without the support of my family and friends, especially my husband's. His endless patience is priceless.

*"We have a unique understanding that most people don't understand
until late in their lives, a perspective learned from critical lessons."*

— Kara Swanson, *I'll Carry the Fork*

Mission

It is my mission to inspire hope and cultivate self-confidence in others struggling with cognitive difficulties by providing practical building blocks for continued rehabilitation after a brain injury. My goal is to create a philosophy of thinking about "how" to do something when a challenge is encountered or a goal is envisioned, enabling survivors to continue their healing process indefinitely.

This guide is the product of what I have learned through my journey as a brain injury survivor and as a result of facilitating brain injury survivor support groups for the Brain Injury Association of Massachusetts since 1995. It incorporates what hundreds of brain injury survivor support group members have learned from their doctors and therapists, countless workshops, conferences, research and most preciously, from each other. It is a collection of "brain injury survivor wisdom".

I am not suggesting that by employing a few strategies from this guide, you will have the magic answer to brain injury recovery. Healing and rehabilitating from a brain injury takes a long time. It continues long after formal rehabilitation has ended. It is the hardest work I have ever done. It requires endless courage, determination, motivation and support. It usually involves rebuilding multiple areas of not just your Life but also your Being – all at once. How could there be an easy solution for all of that!

Brain injury doesn't have to be a destination. It is a journey. Let it be only part of who you are to become.

"Don't accept timetables for recovery."

— Jill Bolte Taylor, PhD, Neuroanatomist

Table of Contents

About the Author: Barbara J. Webster

When a car skidded into mine on a slippery road in 1991, I felt very lucky. Although my car was totaled, I had my seatbelt on and I didn't have a scratch on me. I had blacked out only momentarily and I looked OK! The emergency room sent me home with instructions to take Advil.

I couldn't think because I was exhausted and I was in so much pain. I had a severe case of TMJ or "whiplash". I could barely eat or talk. As I slowly healed and was able to do more physically, I began to realize that I couldn't do anything mentally that I used to do so effortlessly. I was a wife and mother; I managed the household. I had worked professionally in teaching, banking and health care. I was an achiever: multitasking, problem solving and organizing were second nature to me. Now I couldn't remember what I was doing. I couldn't figure out what to wear. I couldn't find my words. I couldn't remember what I was trying to say and if I got interrupted, it was like a train getting derailed, I couldn't get back on track. I couldn't follow the storyline while reading to my son or watching TV. Noise and confusion quickly overloaded and overwhelmed me; like a computer getting too many demands too quickly. But I looked OK!

I had been a home economics and early childhood teacher. Now I couldn't cook supper and I couldn't tolerate the noise and confusion of children. I was a banker and a bank officer and I couldn't hold 2 plus 2 in my head long enough to get 4! I had lived in Framingham for 20 years and I couldn't find my way around. But I looked OK!

My brain used to feel like a fancy multi-function copy machine, copying, sorting and collating all at once. Now, the harder I tried to do what I used to do, the more "meltdowns" and "shutdowns" I had. I thought I was losing my mind and I didn't dare tell anyone. I wasn't feeling so lucky anymore. But I looked OK!

Reality began to set in when I accompanied my son to an evaluation for school. I sat beside him, going through the tests in my head as he answered the questions out loud and I realized that he was doing better on the tests than I was! He was diagnosed with processing and memory problems. He was in second grade. But I was a college graduate!

Cautiously I mentioned this experience to my rheumatologist who had been my doctor for a long time. She said I needed a neuropsychological exam and fought my insurance company for me. Finally, after nine months, I had the testing. I was diagnosed with a "mild" brain injury but I was told I was doing fine - I was figuring out my strategies! Imagine my dismay! During the testing I had related how I had figured out how to do grocery shopping again, a process that now took me 3 days.

I didn't feel like I was doing fine, quite the opposite. I was fighting depression. I had started seeing a counselor and when I asked her if she knew of any help for this diagnosis I had, her response was: "If there is any help, I would think the neuropsychologist who did your testing would have been obligated to tell you about it." I still remember driving home from that appointment, many years ago. I almost lost hope. I thought I was going to go crazy and die. I contemplated suicide.

Fortunately, not too long after that, my son's school featured a speaker from the Brain Injury Association of Massachusetts at a parents' meeting. I had to investigate, even though I rarely had the energy to go out at night. As I sat in the back of the room and listened to this brave survivor speak, tears rolled down my face; finally I was not alone! I approached her after the meeting and she offered to take me to a support group. I was stunned, there is a Brain Injury Association in Massachusetts and there are support groups?! At the support group meeting, as I listened to other survivors tell their stories, I realized that some of these people were getting help, that rehab. wasn't just for people with substance abuse problems and that I didn't have to go crazy and die, literally. Quick, please sign me up! They did sign me up and the therapists helped me begin the long process of putting my life back together.

Meanwhile, I took my husband to a support group meeting and he began to understand that I wasn't getting upset because I was mad at him; I was upset with myself and I had a problem, a BIG problem. During one of those first support group meetings I expressed my frustration about keeping track of what I was doing, even taking a shower! Someone in the group shared the strategy he used to help him remember what he was doing in the shower and it felt like a light came on in my brain! There was a way out of this terrible place I was in; there was HOPE!

Today, my brain can work like that fancy copy machine again - if conditions are optimum. I can do quality work again if I plan it, allowing extra time for fatigue and "bad brain days". I have rebuilt skills and regained stamina. I am able to hear my intuition. Today, I can depend on myself again - if I plan and pace myself. Sometimes, when I am tired or stressed, I have to work like an old-fashioned copier; one page, one step at a time - but I can get the job done!

Today I am a lucky lady. I have had the privilege of facilitating the Brain Injury Survivor Support Group in Framingham since 1995 and I work part time for the Brain Injury Association of Massachusetts assisting other support groups. I get to do something I am passionate about and I get to work with good people. Brain injury survivors and the people who work with them are typically quality people, people who aren't focused on superficial things. Best of all, I get to witness survivors take steps in their healing process and move forward, knowing that my work has helped to play a part in their progress.
What an honor! Today I am a lucky lady!

Introduction
Strategies, Light Bulbs and Hope

It seems to me, before my injury, the connections in my brain were like smooth super highways with information zipping around, sorting and filing almost effortlessly, almost all of the time. Post injury these connections were like roads under major construction, torn up pathways full of obstacles and detours, disconnected. Information tediously struggled to find new pathways and to connect, painfully taking much more time and energy to process, constantly getting stuck or lost. It was frustrating, discouraging, exhausting and mind boggling, just to try to think!

Emerging research on the brain is finally able to validate what we survivors have known all along, that many "roads" or pathways in the brain can be rebuilt and new connections can be made after an injury. Processing information gets smoother and faster with practice, just as traveling around a construction site gets easier in time, as you learn the detour or a new road is made.

Strategies are the key! They are "light bulb moments" for me. Each one is like a little miracle, enabling me to do something I couldn't do otherwise. Strategies give me Hope. The strategies and accommodations described in this guide are suggestions; please modify them to suit your needs. If something you are doing is working for you, don't change it! Every person, every situation and every brain injury is unique. Some skills will be easier to rebuild than others. Most of the suggestions in this guide are not complicated, we just aren't used to thinking that way. We need a different skill set now.

Just glancing at all of these strategies may feel overwhelming and impossible, understandably. It is more work, in a situation that is already overwhelming. Change is hard. You didn't have to do this before. It takes more energy. You are already tired. It can seem like you are going backward and feel like failure. Sometimes it is necessary to take a step backward, in order to take two steps forward.

This guide is intended to assist a wide range of brain injury survivors. Start small, with the chapter that interests you the most. As you figure out what strategies work for you, you will be able to transfer much of what you learn to the next challenge. New challenges will become less scary and less difficult. It won't feel like you are "reinventing the wheel" every time you try to do something.

Many strategies pertain to more than one topic and are worth repeating. If you think you already read something, you probably did! Good memory!

I encourage you to share this guide with family and others in your support system. They can make a big difference in your ability to be comfortable with them by employing a few simple strategies that are helpful to you. My husband developed a habit of saying, "take your time" when he saw me struggling. Hearing this felt like such a gift to me! I would relax a little and be able to figure out what I was doing. If instead he were impatient, I would have felt more stress and had even more difficulty figuring out what I was doing.

Know that in time, as you heal, it won't always be this hard. You won't have to plan and strategize each and every little step you take. So remember you are healing, imagine yourself with a cast on your head and be kind to yourself. Treat yourself like you would any loved one with a serious health issue.

Remember to reward yourself for every successful task and effort, no matter how small. Pat yourself on the back and take a break doing something that will make you smile. We have to be our own cheerleaders now, like the supportive people in our lives were when we were growing up.

Believe In Yourself!

Celebrate Your Successes!

You Can Improve!

The Other Dimension of Brain Injury Healing

Strategies for Rebuilding Self Confidence

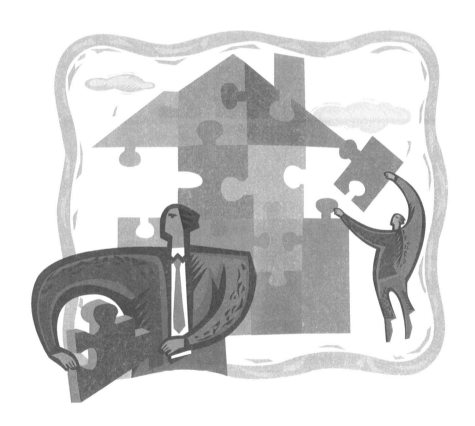

The Other Dimension of Brain Injury Healing

Strategies for Rebuilding Self-Confidence

"If you talk to a man in a language he understands, that goes to his head.
If you talk to him in his language, that goes to his heart."

— Nelson Mandela

Equally as devastating as suddenly losing what seemed like all of my skills and abilities as a result of my brain injury, I was losing all my self-confidence and my sense of self-worth. It was quickly and steadily chipped away every time I tried and couldn't do something that I used to be able to do with such ease. The little things were the most frustrating. Why can't I remember the names of family and friends? Why am I struggling to find every word? Why can't I hold on to my train of thought? Why can't I add 2+2, literally? Why can't I figure out what to wear? Why can't I cook supper? Why do I keep getting lost in the car? Why can't I remember what I am reading? Why can't I remember what I am doing? Why are conversations so difficult to follow? Why can't I follow a plot line on a television show? Why does the sound of the TV make me feel like I want to scream? Why can't I think? Is this what "going crazy" feels like?

Like many of you, I was one of those "achiever people" who defined herself by her accomplishments. When I couldn't do anything I used to be able to do, I felt that my life had no value and I had no reason for being. I was wrong - but it took me some time to figure that out. How do you rebuild self-confidence and a sense of self-worth after they have been devastated?

Discovering strategies gave me Hope and a place to start but it was also absolutely imperative for me to set myself up to succeed as much as possible. My psyche was battered and fragile. It couldn't take any more failure. So I developed a habit of extensive planning, anticipating and strategizing around all possible difficulties. I did this every time I attempted something I hadn't done since my brain injury. It was tedious and time consuming but I began having small successes instead of constant failures. Experiencing small successes began to rebuild my self-confidence.

Developing a sense of self-worth was a little more complicated. If I couldn't do what I used to do, of what value was my life now? I also had no idea I was going through a grieving process. Healing this dimension of brain injury involved profound soul searching and a lot of support from the spiritual guides in my life.

Suggestions for Promoting Emotional Healing

Keep a grateful journal or a victory log

At the end of every day, write down at least three positive things that happened, anything that made you smile or that was an improvement that day. You don't have to write a lot, just a few descriptive words will do.

This simple task can be transforming! It can shift your focus to looking for positive things throughout the day that you can write down in your journal or log at the end of the day. It lifted me out of depression.

Discover your "inner poet"

Write phrases or words that are meaningful to you. The words don't have to rhyme or follow a cadence. Try not to think "I can't" and just start writing whatever comes to mind. If you discover you want to continue, you can type up your poems and make a booklet, adding to it whenever the spirit moves you. It can be for your eyes only or to share with others.

> Tips: Use a pencil with an eraser and lined paper.
> Be sure to date your poems.

When I participated in a poetry workshop with my support group I felt blocked. I didn't think I would write anything, never mind "poetry"! However, once I started, the words just flowed, tapping into emotions that had never been expressed before. It was a similar experience for everyone in the group. It was a profound workshop for all of us and we wanted to write more!

Journaling

If you enjoy writing, journaling can provide another outlet for feelings, as well as perspective when you look back in time. Any writing is also a technique for working on language skills! Writing by hand, with pen or pencil on paper, can help build fine motor skills.

I recommend establishing a time of day to write and writing in your journal every day. Write as little or as much as you feel like writing that day. You can use any notebook, as fancy or as simple as you like. Using something with lined paper and a pencil with an eraser is probably easiest. Be sure to date your pages for future reference.

Please note: I use the word "writing" loosely. Words can be created with pen or pencil, typed on a computer, dictated to a tape recorder or even represented by pictures.

Keep your perspective

Refer to your calendar and journals to look back and note improvements. Make notes and celebrate what you can do now that you couldn't do 6 months or a year ago.

Challenge negative thoughts

Reframe or restructure, look for positive aspects of unpleasant situations. Think "How?" instead of "I can't!" Think, "What can I learn from this situation?"

Take time to smile!

Make time in every day to do something that makes you smile. Schedule it in your planner! Healing from a brain injury is hard work but your life still needs balance or it will become depressing. Surprisingly, doing something you enjoy is energizing!

Forgive yourself

You may not be able to do what you used to do. Remember, you are human.

Remember that you are still the same unique and valuable person inside.

You have the same loves that you had before your injury. No one and no injury can take them away from you!

Be with people who make you feel good about yourself.

You may need to avoid difficult people and situations for the time being. You are healing and you need to be around people who support that process.

Work with art

Use any medium you enjoy!

Do a PhotoVoice Project!

Telling your story with photographs and narratives can be a powerful tool for processing emotions. It is also a wonderful way to work on a variety of skills. Please see the guide in Chapter 16 for Doing Your Own PhotoVoice Project. Expertise in photography is not necessary.

If photography is not your favorite medium, your photos could be created by drawing, painting or even cutting pictures out of magazines and then writing narratives about them.

Grieving Process

I wish I'd known when I was injured that that there is commonly a grieving process associated with healing from a brain injury. You have lost much of your "sense of self". You don't know how much you will get back and you may not know for a long time.

There are often secondary losses as well - jobs, income, homes, friends, even family. These changes and losses can all have a profound effect on a survivor, as well as their family and friends.

It is essential to grieve and mourn the losses in order to heal and move forward. There are general stages associated with the grieving process: denial, anger, bargaining, depression and acceptance. However, healing and processing grief is not a straightforward path. Typically one moves back and forth in the different stages. It is important to know that this is "normal". You can move through them. Support groups can help. Professional help is often necessary. Spiritual guidance may be essential.

Keep in mind that your family members and friends may be grieving too. They have lost the person you used to be and the roles you used to play in their lives. They don't know how much of your former self will return, or when.

"Honoring your feelings is what helps you move beyond the pain."

— Janelle Breese-Biagioni
An Extraordinary Mourning: Understanding Grief after a Brain Injury

If you are having trouble believing in yourself or are losing hope, please seek professional help and get in touch with your spiritual guides, whatever and whomever they may be.

Preventing Shutdown and Meltdowns

Strategies for
Managing Fatigue and Overload

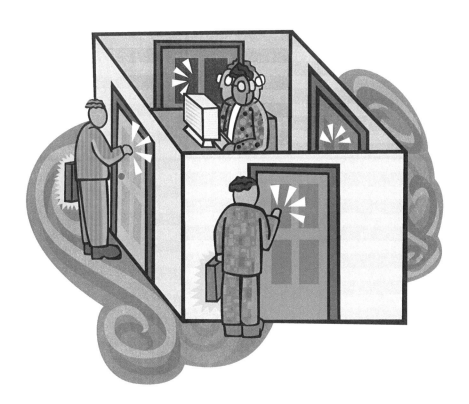

Preventing Shutdown and Meltdowns

Strategies for Managing Fatigue and Overload

"Being a brain injury survivor = Being a stranger in a familiar place."

— Beverly Bryant
In Search of Wings

Many brain injury survivors experience a "brain fatigue" unlike anything they have ever experienced before. Your brain feels fatigued long before your body. You feel overloaded, overwhelmed and stressed to the breaking point. You can't think. Your brain feels foggy, lost, stuck or blocked. It feels like there is a "logjam" in your "river" of thoughts. It is exasperating, exhausting and depressing. In addition, you probably have pain and fatigue from your physical injuries. Balancing and pacing are key for your brain as well as your body. The challenge is to find your new healthy balance.

Before your injury, you had a pool of reserve energy that you could draw from when you overextended yourself. You were likely able to give 110% at times. After a brain injury, nearly all your energy may be needed just to simply function. You are not able to push beyond 100%, no matter how much you want to. There is no reserve. When you push yourself too much, you feel overwhelmed and overloaded. It can cause setbacks. It can cause irrational behavior. It can make you physically ill.

Remember you are healing, even if you can't see a wound! Think of your brain in a cast, as it would be if you broke any other part of your body. If you broke your leg, you wouldn't expect yourself to run a marathon right away, even if you were previously a marathon runner. First you would be in a cast and you would rest a lot. Then you would start walking with crutches on even surfaces. The next step might be walking with a cane. You get the idea; it would take a lot of healing before you could run again, never mind run a marathon! Most of us try to run marathons with our brains all the time!

You won't be able to do everything you used to, at least not right away. Everything will be harder and take a lot longer to do than it used to. You can compensate by cutting back, simplifying and being kind and patient with yourself. Avoid the tendency to push yourself too hard. Rehabilitation is a delicate balance between challenging yourself enough to promote healing and not so much that you have discouraging setbacks.

So picture yourself with a cast on your head and remember to rest, celebrate the smallest gains and balance out all the hard work with something that makes you smile, every day. You are engaged in one of the toughest challenges of your life, if not *the* hardest but it will get easier in time.

17

Practical Suggestions

<u>Do what you can to get a good night's sleep.</u>

<u>If you can't sleep, you can't recharge and heal.</u>

- ❏ Maintain regular sleep schedules, going to bed and getting up at the same time each day.
- ❏ Try not to nap for more than 1 hour or after 3:00 p.m.
- ❏ Take pain medication as prescribed.
- ❏ Get some exercise every day.
- ❏ Avoid getting overtired.
- ❏ Limit caffeine.
- ❏ Avoid heavy meals and exercise late in the day.
- ❏ Plan "down time" before bedtime.

Please note: Brain injury often disrupts normal sleep patterns. If these suggestions don't help, consult your doctor or a sleep specialist.

<u>Maintain a healthy diet.</u>

Your body and your brain need substance to function.

<u>Don't stand when you can sit. Don't sit when you can lie down.</u>

For example, cut up vegetables while sitting at the table instead of standing at the sink. Fold laundry while sitting instead of standing. Lie down or recline in a chair to watch TV or rest.

<u>Simplify your life.</u>

Eliminate as many "must dos" as possible and make things as easy on yourself as possible, to give you more energy for healing. Lower your expectations. Let it be OK to have simpler meals, use paper plates and cups, wash the towels and sheets less often, skip reading the magazines and junk mail, participate in fewer social activities, let others help you. (See Chapter 12 for more ideas to simplify your life.)

Your personal best is not going to be the same as when you were healthy but it is still your personal best.

<u>Let it be OK to ask for and accept help.</u>

Delegate what you can. This may be very hard for you; it was for me. I felt like a failure. Try to think of it as giving others an opportunity to feel useful. Most people who care about you really want to help. Children can learn valuable skills by helping with daily tasks like meals and laundry, as well as take pride in feeling helpful.

<u>Watch for symptoms of fatigue.</u>

Warning signs include:

- ❏ Increased mistakes
- ❏ Feeling "stuck" or blocked
- ❏ Increased pain
- ❏ Feeling edgy or anxious
- ❏ Increased sensitivities to light
- ❏ Increased sensitivities to sounds

<u>Pushing too hard and overdoing will work against you.</u>

It can cause setbacks; increased pain, fatigue, brain "shutdown" and sometimes "meltdowns". You will end up needing unplanned recuperation time to compensate. This can become very discouraging.

This will probably be especially difficult for you if you are an "achiever". That's because the skills you need now to heal successfully, like pacing and resting, seem to contradict the skills that helped you become successful before your injury, like pushing yourself to complete tasks. You need a new skill set now. This means finding your new limits and working out a healthy balance for a successful day.

<u>The more complex the task, the greater the need for pacing and taking breaks.</u>

You will probably be surprised at how much better you are able to think after a break. This is now a "strategy for success" that may have seemed counter-productive before. If a break doesn't help, then it is time to change to an easier task or stop for the day.

A nap or an extended break can be especially helpful after a big task, before the kids get home from school or before you need to prepare supper. Just try not to nap for more than 1 hour or after 3:00pm.

<u>Figure out what your "best brain time" of day is.</u>

Arrange your day to do your most challenging tasks at that time.

<u>Plan to do tasks that require concentration in a quiet environment with limited distractions, interruptions and interfering sounds.</u>

They all use brain energy. Let the answering machine get the phone. Try putting in earplugs or play some soothing music if background sounds are bothering you. Sometimes it can be helpful to work at the library. Postpone the task if necessary, rather than put yourself in a no-win position.

Work on one task at a time, one step at a time.

Dividing your attention and multi-tasking create stress and drain your energy. They also inhibit memory.

Examples:

❏ Help your children with their homework and <u>then</u> cook supper, perhaps while they watch TV.

❏ When preparing meals, <u>first</u> set the table, <u>second</u> make the salad and <u>third</u> start cooking.

❏ Try not to do anything else while you are on the phone or watching TV.

Slow down, work at your own pace.

Rushing creates stress. It is an energy drain and inhibits memory.

Use good computer posture to minimize pain and fatigue.

You may need to consult an occupational or physical therapist.

Plan your deadlines.

Mark your calendar a few days to a week ahead of the actual deadline to get the bills paid on time, forms filled out, etc. This will allow for pacing and "bad brain days" and minimize stress.

Avoid sensory overload.

It takes brain energy to screen out distractions, confusion, noises and interruptions. <u>You will tire more quickly in busy environments.</u> Plan to limit your exposure to restaurants, parties, crowds and sporting events, etc.

Special events

You will need to be very selective about social activities. They will use up a lot more of your energy than they used to. Think twice before you commit to anything. You might respond by saying, "Can I think about that?" or "I'll have to get back to you about that," or "I wish I could but I just can't right now." No further explanation is needed.

If you decide to participate, figure out how to make the event as easy as possible on yourself. Can you bring something instead of making something? Can you limit the time you are there? Do you have an "escape plan" in case you start to feel overwhelmed and overloaded? Plan an easy day ahead of a big event and a recuperation day afterward.

Pacing and Balancing

Try to think in terms of managing your energy, instead of managing your time. Resist adding that one more thing to the day or to the week when you know deep down inside it will be too much.

- ❏ Learn to recognize your limits, when you aren't working as efficiently anymore.
- ❏ Plan "brain breaks" between tasks – a rest break, a water break, a healthy snack break, a stress management/relaxation break, a change to a physical activity break.
- ❏ Think of naps as "performance strategy". Plan afternoon "downtime" or a short nap, every day.
- ❏ Figure out how many appointments you can handle in a day, without feeling overloaded.
- ❏ Figure out how many days of appointments you can handle in a week, without causing setbacks.

Managing Stress

You can't think well and memory is impaired when you are under stress, especially after a brain injury. Discover your best tools for managing stress and try to think of stress management as a performance strategy.

Exercise, exercise, exercise!

Exercise is a wonderful cure for stress. Just about any form of motion helps relieve tension. If you have mobility or balance issues, chair exercises can be very effective. Activities like yoga, Tai Chi, Qui Gong and repetitive exercises such as running or rowing are all excellent ways to relieve stress. A mindful walk, dancing or even house cleaning for some, can leave you feeling calmer and more centered. Do what you enjoy and remember to pace yourself, even 10 minutes can be helpful. (See Chapter 15 for more on the benefits of exercise.)

What else can you do to turn off your stress engine?

Make a list of things you love to do and observe a daily wind-down period. Some possibilities:

- ❏ Meditation
- ❏ Visualization
- ❏ Slow deep breathing from your diaphragm
- ❏ Give yourself a mini massage
- ❏ Schedule social time
- ❏ Talk to a friend
- ❏ Spend time with your pet
- ❏ Soak in a tub
- ❏ Eat a little chocolate or comfort food
- ❏ Sip chamomile tea

- ❏ Aromatherapy – lavender or any scent you find pleasing
- ❏ Watch a burning candle, crackling fire, lava lamp, fish tank
- ❏ Curl up with a book
- ❏ Listen to music
- ❏ Shout or sing loudly
- ❏ Dance to music
- ❏ Rent a favorite movie
- ❏ Watch a funny television show

Managing Overload and Preventing Meltdowns

Fatigue, pain and pushing yourself beyond your limits can all contribute to meltdowns. They are not pretty. They are always regrettable. They cause setbacks. They can be mistaken for mental health problems.

Learn your signs of overload or neuro-distress.

They may not be clear to you at first but common signs include:

- ❏ Face turning red
- ❏ Distractibility
- ❏ Dizziness
- ❏ Increased pain
- ❏ Heart beating faster
- ❏ Clenched teeth
- ❏ Tightened fists
- ❏ Feeling anxious or edgy
- ❏ Nausea
- ❏ Heightened sensitivities to light or sound
- ❏ Difficulty hearing
- ❏ Trouble focusing
- ❏ Blurred vision

Ask a family member or close friend to help you monitor your stress levels.

You can establish a subtle sign or code word between the two of you that reminds you to check in with how you are feeling. Do this before you feel overwhelmed and unable to deal with the situation appropriately.

TAKE A BREAK when you first notice signs of overload.

Resist that natural tendency to push beyond your limits, like you were able to do before your injury. If you feel like you are going to cry, throw a fit, yell, swear, have a temper tantrum, turn into the "Tasmanian Devil" or get physical in any way – Walk Away!!

Excuse yourself, go to a quiet place (even the bathroom) - close your eyes and do some slow deep breathing, expanding your stomach and counting to seven with each inhale and each exhale. If you continue what you are doing you may go beyond your "point of no return", when it feels like a switch is flipped and you are out of control, having a meltdown.

Try to identify the cause of the meltdown should you have one.

Does it tend to follow any pattern? Are you getting tired or feeling overwhelmed? Is the environment noisy and confusing? Are you trying to do too much? The more you know about what caused it, the better you will be able to respond in a constructive manner and avoid situations that contribute to it.

Be sure to apologize to the people who have been affected by your meltdown.

Apologies demonstrate an awareness of your behavior and go a long way in helping others understand your situation.

Setbacks can be helpful.

They are almost necessary for learning your limits - but you want to minimize them as much as possible. Constant setbacks are depressing. Strive to be able to predict and prevent them as much as possible.

Parenting Tips for School Vacations

When you are a parent with a brain injury, even anticipating school vacations can send you into panic mode. Parenting is such an important job, but it is usually a major challenge just to manage children after school and on weekends. What do you do when you suddenly need to be a full time parent and it is difficult to be around the noise, activity level and confusion that children bring with them? This was one of my biggest challenges as a parent with a brain injury.

Suggestions

Nurture yourself **before** the school vacation.

Set aside a day to do something for YOU. Get that haircut you've been putting off. Treat yourself to a massage or a manicure. Get together with a friend. Go fishing. Pamper yourself a little, so you are recharged and can better handle the challenge ahead.

Surrender to the situation.

Keep things as simple as possible for the duration of the vacation. Postpone any extra projects. This is not the time to reorganize the kitchen cabinets or fix that leaking faucet.

Plan regular breaks for yourself.

If you need a rest break to get through the day when the kids aren't home all day, you're *really* going to need it now. Maybe your rest break can be every afternoon while the kids watch a video. If it is going to be hard for you to resist using that time to catch up on housework, try engaging the kids in a 15-minute clean up first and make movie time a reward - for everyone!

Talk with the kids about the plans for the day.

"After breakfast, we're going to do _____."

"After lunch, there will be time for _____."

"This afternoon we're going to _____."

<u>Plan activities outside of the house.</u>

It doesn't have to be a big deal, even just an hour outside of the house. Changing the environment will be stimulating and help the children settle down when they are home.

- ❏ Local libraries often have programs for children during school vacations.
- ❏ Libraries also have free tickets for local museums and zoos.
- ❏ Area museums often offer a variety of art classes.
- ❏ Churches sometimes have summer programs.
- ❏ Check out community recreation programs, swimming lessons and any other activities that interest your child.
- ❏ Physical activities can be especially beneficial for your children and you! They get to do something they like and you get a break while they participate. They will be ready for a rest period when they get home!
- ❏ Camp can be a lifesaver!
- ❏ If your children grumble about "family time", try not to take it too seriously. They usually have fun once they are engaged. Afterwards they can do something they want to do.

<u>Ask for help.</u>

This is probably the most important advice I can give you. Set yourself up to succeed. Don't try to handle it all yourself if you know in your gut that you probably can't because you are already having enough trouble getting through the weekends when the family is home. Having a break to look forward to can help you get through the more taxing times.

- ❏ Can a spouse take some vacation time and help out by taking the kids to do something while you take a break?
- ❏ Can a relative help out by taking the kids for a few hours?
- ❏ Can you hire a "mother's helper" to supervise the children while you do something else or take a break? Maybe there is an older neighbor child who enjoys your children and would love to earn a few dollars.
- ❏ Can you hire a sitter for a few hours each day or for a couple of afternoons a week?

<u>Try to resist feeling like you need to participate in everything.</u>

You won't get the break you need. Your present reality is that you can't do as much as you used to do. You may miss an experience but if you get the rest you need, your family will have a good experience with you when they return. That might not happen if you are too tired.

Reward yourself for every day you navigate successfully! Write about it in your journal or victory log. Stock up on a favorite treat before the vacation and have a little each night. Know that your tolerances and stamina can increase in time.

Give yourself a BIG reward every time you prevent Overload, Shutdown or a Meltdown!! You can get better at noticing your triggers in time.

Know that tolerances and stamina can improve! In time you can learn your new healthy balance of work and rest. You will be able to do more without causing yourself setbacks.

If you continue to experience extraordinary fatigue, be sure to mention it to your doctor.

A physical therapist or an occupational therapist may be helpful in figuring out how to incorporate some of the strategies mentioned in this chapter.

Keep in mind that your brain injury may have reduced your tolerances to alcohol and medications. So restrict your use of alcohol and check with your doctor to determine if any of the medications you are taking may cause fatigue or agitation as a side effect.

Caps, Sunglasses and Earplugs

Strategies for Coping with Sensory Hypersensitivities

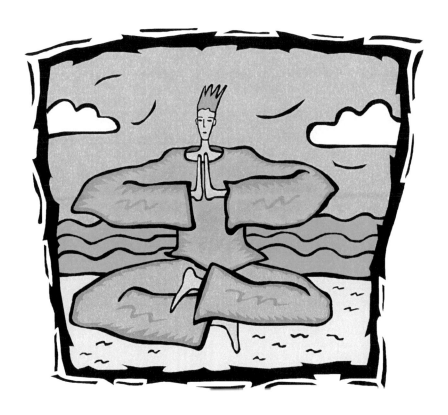

28

Caps, Sunglasses and Earplugs

Strategies for Coping with Sensory Hypersensitivities

"Just as the tumultuous chaos of a thunderstorm brings a nurturing rain that allows life to flourish, so too in human affairs times of advancement are preceded by times of disorder. Success comes to those who can weather the storm."

— I CHING no.3

If it seems like your sense of touch, taste, smell, hearing or vision is extra sensitive or heightened after your brain injury, it's not your imagination. Sensory hypersensitivities are another major, yet not as obvious, contributor to fatigue and overload after brain injury. What we experience with our senses is essentially more information for our injured brains to try to process and organize. You can have difficulties processing sensory information just like any other information in your brain. Some examples of sensory hypersensitivities are:

❑ Sounds that you barely noticed before are alarming and startle you.

❑ It feels like you have megaphones in your ears.

❑ Background sounds and stimulating environments become overwhelming.

❑ Fluorescent and bright lights give you headaches.

❑ Clothing that was comfortable before feels irritating now.

❑ Large gatherings of people feel overwhelming.

Pain and fatigue can intensify sensory hypersensitivities, putting you in a hyper-sensitive or hyper-vigilant state. When you are in a hyper-sensitive or hyper-vigilant state, even subtle stimulants feel overwhelming. Especially sights and sounds that didn't bother you before, may now trigger anxiety and the fight-or-flight response where your whole being feels threatened and out of control. You may shut down and not be able to do any more or you may feel compelled to escape from the situation. It can be very taxing, physically and mentally.

Stress management, movement and using <u>all</u> of your senses can help your brain organize and integrate the senses. This is similar to what children do. Consider how physically active children are as they grow and develop!

See ***Brain Recharging Breaks*** at the end of this chapter for some basic meditation techniques. Meanwhile, following are suggestions for coping with sensory hypersensitivities.

General Coping Suggestions

<u>Limit exposure to avoid sensory overload.</u>

❏ Avoid crowds and chaotic places where there are a lot of stimuli, like shopping malls.

❏ Do shopping and errands early in the week and early in the day, when stores are less crowded and quieter.

❏ Shop in smaller, quieter stores when possible.

❏ Eat out in restaurants when they are quieter, in between regular meal times.

❏ Hold conversations in a quiet place.

❏ Ask people to please speak one at a time. Explain that you'd really like to hear what everyone has to say but you can only hear one person at a time.

❏ Sleep during car trips.

❏ If you want to attend a function that you expect will be taxing, <u>plan</u> to stay only a short while. Take your cap, sunglasses and earplugs. Sit towards the back to minimize the sound and where you can easily exit to a quieter place or the car.

<u>Monitor your pain, stress and fatigue levels.</u>

Lights and sounds will bother you the most when you are stressed or fatigued. If you are feeling especially sensitive, use it as a cue that you need to take a break and use some relaxation techniques.

<u>Try avoiding nicotine, caffeine and alcohol.</u>

They may make the symptoms worse. If you have vertigo, try limiting your salt intake, which can cause fluid retention. Consider strengthening exercises for your neck with the guidance of a physical therapist.

<u>When you are starting to feel stressed or anxious, try incorporating another sense.</u>

❏ Put something in your mouth to chew or suck on. Strong flavors like peppermint or cinnamon are especially effective.

❏ Put on some soothing music.

❏ Apply some deep pressure. Give yourself a hug or press your palms firmly together or on the table. Squeeze the steering wheel if you are driving the car.

<u>Experiment with activities and alternative therapies that involve your senses.</u>

Listen to music, experiment with movement, dance, yoga, water, art, aromatherapy, etc.

<u>Challenge your sensitivities.</u>

Gradually increase your exposure and tolerance when using earplugs, sunglasses, etc. *Don't eliminate the senses completely or you set yourself up for super-sensitivity.*

Specific Coping Strategies

Sensitivities to sound

❏ Limit your exposure to noisy stores and loud situations like sporting events, the movie theatre and children's school activities. Don't participate or plan to stay for a limited amount of time. Sit on the outskirts so you can gracefully escape to a quieter place if needed.

❏ Use earplugs, try different kinds, and carry them with you.

❏ Use headphones for TV and music:
  - For others, when you don't want to hear it.
  - For yourself, when you want to hear it better.

❏ Minimize distractions from snacking while doing things like working in groups or playing games. Use bowls for food instead of eating directly from noisy bags.

❏ Add some background sound – a fan, white noise machine, soothing music.

❏ Remove yourself from the situation and go to a quieter place as soon as possible, even the bathroom, when you feel overwhelmed or anxious. Then try:
  - Closing your eyes
  - Taking slow deep stomach breaths
  - Putting an ice pack on your forehead and eyes

❏ Gradually expose yourself to different sounds and louder sounds to increase your tolerances.

Sensitivities to light

❏ Avoid bright light and fluorescent lights.

❏ Use sunglasses or a cap with a brim, even indoors.

❏ Try yellow tinted glasses if florescent lights are a problem.

❏ Try polarized sunglasses if driving glare is a problem.

❏ Try yellow tinted glasses if night driving is a problem.

❏ Make sure you are getting plenty of vitamin A (but not too much!).

❏ Eat orange colored fruits and vegetables like carrots, sweet potatoes, squash and cantaloupe.

❏ Take a moment to just close your eyes for a few minutes when you are starting to feel stressed or anxious. This blocks out the visual stimuli.

<u>Sensitivities to touch, taste and smell</u>

- ❏ Experiment! Cultivate an awareness of how things feel, taste and smell.
- ❏ Rub different textures on your arms, increasing the intensity to gradually decrease sensitivities.
- ❏ Add texture, contrasting temperatures and flavors to your food, like ice cream with crunchy nuts or chips with spicy taco sauce.
- ❏ Notice the textures.
- ❏ Pay attention to smells.
- ❏ How do different aromas make you feel?

If your sense of smell is altered, make sure to have functioning smoke and gas detectors in your home.

<u>Doing cognitive work</u>

- ❏ Plan to do cognitive work when your environment is quiet. Eliminate as many distractions and interruptions as possible.
- ❏ Screen out distractions by using earplugs or headphones, playing soothing music, or using a fan or white noise machine if you have sensitivities to sound.
- ❏ Turn down the volume on the phone and let the machine get it.
- ❏ Work in an uncluttered space or use a three sided table screen, to help screen out visual distractions.
- ❏ Give children headphones for the TV if you are having trouble screening it out.
- ❏ Do your "thinking" work while children are in school or asleep.
- ❏ Still having trouble concentrating? Try bringing in another sense.
  - ○ Put on some soothing nature or instrumental music, something without words at a low volume.
  - ○ Try chewing or sucking on something while you are working. Coffee stirrers can substitute for fingernails. Strong flavored or fizzy candies and gum can aid alertness.
  - ○ Try using some deep pressure by giving yourself a hug, pressing your palms strongly against each other or on the table.
  - ○ Try sitting on a large therapy ball while you work. A great strategy if you have trouble sitting still!
- ❏ Take a physical break, every 15 min. at first. *Resist the urge to push through.* I know it feels counter-intuitive but taking breaks will actually help you work longer! Gradually you will find you can increase the time between breaks.
  - ○ Use a timer - without a ticking sound!
  - ○ Pause and stretch, drink some water or make a cup of tea, walk around the house or the yard, rock in a chair, walk the dog, pat the cat.

Visual Processing Problems

Vision is an extremely important and complex source of sensory information. What you see with your eyes travels through your brain to the back area of your brain, where it is processed in the occipital lobe. There is a lot of territory between the eyes and the back of the brain where an injury can occur. The occipital lobe may be damaged directly from impact to the back of the head or it may be damaged indirectly from the ricochet of the brain inside the skull when the front of the brain is impacted. Damage to the occipital lobe frequently occurs in car accidents, falls and sports injuries. Even subtle visual problems following a brain injury can have a significant impact on cognition and functioning.

I wish I had known about visual problems and visual therapy when I had my car accident. I thought I was really going crazy! Fortunately for me, my issues improved with time but not without mishaps, like falling off a curb!

Some common problems after a brain injury related to vision include:

- ❏ Double vision
- ❏ Trouble tracking words on a page
- ❏ Impaired depth perception
- ❏ Hypersensitivities to light
- ❏ Difficulties remembering and recalling information that is seen
- ❏ Difficulties "filling in the gaps" or completing a picture based on seeing only some of the parts
- ❏ Trouble seeing objects to the side
- ❏ Low tolerances to changing light or clutter
- ❏ Impaired balance, bumping into objects
- ❏ Feeling overwhelmed when there is a lot of visual stimuli

If you notice problems in areas related to visual processing, please consult a visual therapist or a neuroopthalmologist, they can help!

Tips:

- ❏ Don't eliminate any sense completely or you set yourself up for a super-sensitivity.
- ❏ Gradually expose yourself to more light, sound, touch, smell and taste.
- ❏ Be patient, in many cases your sensory hypersensitivities will decrease in time!
- ❏ Ask for physical therapy or occupational therapy with a therapist with a background in sensory integration for help with sensory sensitivities.

Some good news about sensory hypersensitivity is that it is also associated with a heightened sense of awareness and intuition. You may find that you feel more aware of your intuition and more creative since your brain injury. This is not uncommon. Enjoy!

Brain Recharging Breaks

If I had to choose one strategy that helped me the most after my brain injury, it would be learning to meditate. Meditation is especially helpful when you are experiencing sensory overload. It can help you calm yourself down from that hyper-sensitive state. It was also the only way I have found to give my brain a rest, to put it temporarily in a "cast", like you would a broken limb. Often, after meditating for 15-20 minutes, the "logjam" in my brain clears up and I am somehow able to think again!

I recommend using some stress management or meditation techniques at least once a day. <u>Plan it</u>, schedule it in your planner, make it part of your daily routine. Meditation is not as mysterious as you might think. Try these basic steps:

- ❏ Get in a comfortable position on the bed, in a recliner or even in the car; uncross your arms and legs. Cover yourself with a blanket if you are cool.
- ❏ Close your eyes and do some slow deep breathing.
- ❏ Slowly inhale, expanding your stomach and counting to 7.
- ❏ Exhale gradually, contracting your stomach towards your spine, counting to 7.

Repeat. Repeat. Repeat.

When you are feeling more relaxed, as you continue your slow deep breathing, experiment with the following suggestions to increase the effectiveness of the experience.

Do a body scan checking for areas of pain or stress.

- ❏ Eyes closed, inhale deeply, picture your forehead and notice any stress or pain.
- ❏ Exhale and imagine the pain floating away with your exhale.
- ❏ Inhale, picture your eyebrows and notice any stress or pain. Exhale and release it, imagining the stress floating away.
- ❏ Repeat for your eyes, ears, jaw, throat, back of neck, shoulders … down to your toes. Breathe in relaxation, breathe out stress and pain.

Notice how you feel after you get to your toes!

- ❏ Visualize or imagine yourself in a warm, secure, relaxing, happy, peaceful place; floating on a cloud, floating in the water, or recalling a happy memory.
  - ○ Continue slow deep breathing.
- ❏ Focus on a picture or artwork that you like, noticing each detail.
  - ○ Continue slow deep breathing.
- ❏ Listen to music, any music that is soothing to you. Nature sounds or instrumental music is a good place to start experimenting.
  - ○ Continue slow deep breathing.
- ❏ Use aromatherapy – any scent that smells good to you. Favorite scents are often from childhood memories!
  - ○ Continue slow deep breathing.

Tools

Strive to let go of that never-ending tape of worries and "shoulds" that plays in your head. Focus on your senses – your breath, the music, a relaxing place, a comforting aroma. If thoughts drift in, gently push them away. It gets easier with practice, you'll find what works best for you and you'll be amazed at how much it helps you!

If you find these suggestions helpful and you want to learn more, check out classes in meditation, yoga, Tai Chi and Qui Gong. Local medical facilities and high schools often offer classes at reasonable rates.

There are television programs that demonstrate different practices as well as a variety of DVDs you can rent from your local library to get an idea of which discipline suits you best.

More Than Writing It Down

Strategies for Improving Memory

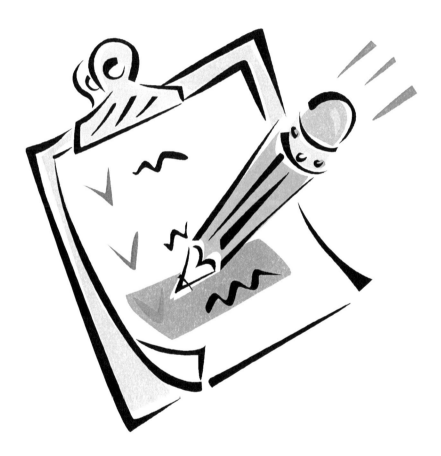

More Than Writing It Down

Strategies for Improving Memory

"I felt a cleavage in my mind as if my brain had split;
I tried to match it, seam by seam, but could not make them fit.
The thought behind I strove to join unto the thought before,
But sequence raveled out of reach like balls upon a floor."

— Emily Dickinson

It is helpful to keep in mind that there are two basic categories of memory processing:

1. **Recall**

   This involves retrieving information *from* the brain.
   The information is already stored in memory.

2. **Registration**

   This involves getting information *into* the brain. It is also referred to as imprinting, encoding, storing and learning. This is a common problem for survivors of brain injury. While it may seem that you can't recall or remember well, much of the problem may actually be due to difficulties storing or registering information in your brain.

So, Recall of new information is dependent on Registration.
If the information doesn't get registered in the brain, it can't be recalled!

Suggestions for Improving Memory Registration

Establish routines for daily tasks.

For example, your routine for getting up each and every morning might be:

❏ Wake up
❏ Take a.m. pills
❏ Shower
❏ Brush teeth, shave
❏ Get dressed
❏ Comb hair
❏ Make bed
❏ Prepare and eat breakfast
❏ Check planner/calendar

Repeating the steps in the same order or sequence every morning will help the steps become more and more automatic and easier to remember. It may be helpful to make a list of your steps and post it in your bedroom.

Make notes on the spot.

Use a pocket recorder or the message feature on your cell phone/electronic organizer when it is not convenient to write things down. For example, make a note where you parked your car or to remember to pick something up at the grocery store on your way home.

Keep track of medications.

Use pillboxes that can be set up for the day or the week, whatever works best for you.

Medication reminders

Use an alarm on your watch/cell phone/electronic organizer to help you remember when to take your medications.

Appointment reminders

Use an alarm on your watch/cell phone/electronic organizer for appointment reminders. Consider travel time and set the alarm for **the time you need to leave** in order to arrive at the appointment on time.

Link a new activity with an established routine.

For example, take morning medications when you brush your teeth. Check your planner when you have your morning coffee.

Talk to yourself (quietly) as you do things.

This practice can help your language skills as well as your memory recall.

<u>Write it down!</u>

Write down what is important in your life. (Try not to fall into the trap of writing *everything* down; it can be counter-productive.) Just the act of writing something down enhances your ability to remember it. Having things in writing reduces the amount of retrieval your brain needs to do. It also creates a memory tool. Examples:

❑ Write up your medical history.
> Keep it in your planner or appointment folder, whatever you always take with you to medical appointments. This is especially helpful when you see a new health care provider. You will need to update it periodically. (Sample at end of chapter.)

❑ Post a list of frequently dialed phone numbers.
> Organize it by category and have it near your phone at home to use when you are there. If you program numbers into your phone and never dial them, you will not re-learn them and you will have a big problem if your phone is lost. (Template at end of chapter.)

❑ Keep a small notebook and pencil beside the phone for messages.
> Loose paper can easily get misplaced.

❑ Use a telephone log.
> This helps track ongoing issues and correspondence like insurance and billing problems. (Sample at end of chapter.)

❑ Make a cueing and reminder system for yourself.
> To remember information about family and friends, you can keep notes and questions for future calls in your address book.

❑ Create lists.
> Lists are invaluable memory tools. When you review them at the end of the day, it may surprise you how much you actually did get done!

> Examples of lists:
>> <u>Checklists for routines</u>; your morning routine, leaving the kitchen, before you go to bed, paying bills, etc. (Sample "Getting Out the Door Checklist" at end of chapter.)

>> <u>Memory Jogger Lists</u>, lists of issues to consider for "To Do" Lists. (Sample at end of chapter.)

>> <u>"To Do" Lists,</u> for the day, paperwork to be done, for errands, groceries, shopping, etc.

Please refer to the Chapter 7 on Organization for more details about lists.

Repetitions, repetitions, repetitions

Repetition is the foundation of the rehabilitation process. The pathways in your brain get stronger and more efficient with each repetition. Repetitions also give you an opportunity to note improvement with each repetition!

Take advantage of opportunities to repeat doing things such as:

- ❏ Listening to phone messages as many times as you need to
- ❏ Reading and rereading material
- ❏ Recording and watching a favorite television show again
- ❏ Watching a movie more than once
- ❏ Attending the same workshop more than once
- ❏ Auditing a class before you take it
- ❏ Taking dry runs in the car to find new locations

Work on one task at a time, one step at a time and work at your own pace.

By doing this, whatever you do will register better in your brain. For example:

- ❏ Don't try to answer the phone or help children with homework while you are cooking.

- ❏ Don't try to do anything else while you are on the phone or watching TV if you want to remember what you are doing.

- ❏ Try to work deliberately, at a pace that feels comfortable for you. Working too fast for your brain to keep up and register or store what you are doing will start to feel very confusing.

- ❏ When checking your work, check one task at a time. For example, when I check what I have written; first, I read it over to make sure it makes sense, then I spell-check, then I check formatting and spacing. If I tried to check everything at the same time, I would lose track of what I was checking and become confused.

Use all your senses when you want to remember something.

Notice how something looks, sounds, smells and feels when you are doing something. You are creating a stronger memory for recall.

Use physical cues.

- ❏ Try playing indoor basketball or rocking in a chair while you are practicing something you need to remember. Some of us process information better when we are physically engaged.

- ❏ Try sitting on a therapy ball while you are doing important desk work if it is hard for you to sit still.

- ❏ Try standing on one foot, close to something you can grab for balance if you need to, while repeating to yourself what you want to remember. Throwing yourself slightly off balance will bring your body to alert and help you remember.

Use visual cues.

❏ Label cabinets and drawers to help you remember where things are.

❏ Post sticky notes and checklists – on your mirror, by the front door, in the car, etc, wherever it is useful. Use different colors for different activities. Change the color or location of the lists periodically so you don't start screening them out and not seeing them. Remove them when you don't need them anymore.

❏ Post a photo, instead of a list, of the items you need to remember when you leave the house.

❏ Place items where you will see them when you need them.

Examples:

o Place your medications where you will see them when you need to take the medication; on your dresser, near the kitchen sink or on the kitchen table (and keep them out of the reach of children and pets).

o Make designated places for items that you use daily like eyeglasses and keys, <u>on top of</u> the table instead of inside a drawer.

o Keep your planner or organizer, cell phone, wallet or purse, keys and driving glasses near the front door where you will see them when you leave the house. You might even need to pile things in front of the door to help you see them!

Note: If you are always misplacing your keys, try clipping them to your purse or belt loop or on a cord around your neck.

o Keep your files where you can see them and near where you need to use them. Items will be more likely to get filed!

❏ Place the materials for whatever you need to work on that day on the table - planner, folders, grocery list, bills, etc. They will serve as cues for what you want to do that day. Be sure to use a table that won't be disturbed by others. As you complete the job put the materials away.

❏ Prepare for appointments. Make a list of questions to ask before the appointment. Put the list in your planner or a folder and place it near your keys and wallet to help you remember to take it with you.

Suggestions for Improving Memory Recall

<u>Check your planner/organizer or calendar and "To Do" Lists first thing in the morning!</u>

Make it a habit so you don't miss something important.

<u>Check your Memory Jogger Lists before you begin tasks!</u>

<u>Establish designated places for important items.</u>

… like eyeglasses, medications, car keys, wallet/purse, etc. Always put them away in the same place, then you will know where to find them.

<u>Feeling "blocked" trying to remember a word?</u>

- ❏ Try describing or defining the word:
    - ○ "The thing that changes the channels on the television" = the REMOTE!
    - ○ "The things that keep my hands warm" = GLOVES!
    - ○ "The blue and white thing that goes on my head" = HAT!
    - ○ Ask if the person you are talking to can think of the word you are trying to remember. The person may enjoy helping you figure it out.
    - ○ If you are writing, a thesaurus can be a huge frustration saver.

<u>Having trouble remembering something when you are listening to someone?</u>

Explain that you are having trouble remembering what they are talking about. Ask the person if they could tell you more about it. When did it happen? Where did it take place. Who else was there?

<u>Remembering people and situations you haven't been in since your injury</u>

It could be very helpful to look at photos or read material about the subject to refresh your memory, before the meeting, like you might do for a class reunion.

<u>Feeling "blocked" or stuck trying to recall a place, event or situation?</u>

Try using your senses. Visualize the situation. Where were you? Who else was there? What time of day was it? What was the weather like? What did it sound like? What did it smell like? Can you ask someone to describe it? Can you look back at your journal, calendar or photo albums to help frame the situation?

<u>If you find yourself not remembering what you are doing –</u>

… like where you are going when you are in the car - are you tired or hungry or distracted and not fully focused on what you are doing? You could be preoccupied with thoughts, rushing and trying to attend to too many things at the same time. Information may not be registering in your brain. Take a break. Drink some water, have a snack, refer to your list or planner.

<u>Take notes if you find yourself losing track of what is being said at a meeting or a lecture.</u>

Use key words and "topic specific" doodles or sketches to create memory cues. You can also use a tape recorder, just remember to ask permission.

<u>It's OK **not** to remember everything.</u>

In our very busy world, even the most accomplished people use memory aids. If you can't remember something, don't make it up. It will only cause more confusion. Forgive yourself for not being "Perfect." Get in the habit of saying things that give you time to think and remember, like "Let me think about that" or "I'll have to check on that" or "Can I get back to you on that?"

> *"Acknowledging successes helps build self-confidence.*
> *Self-confidence is the number-one memory builder."*

> — Dennis P. Swiercinsky,
> *50 Ways You Can Improve Your Memory*

<u>Helpful tips …</u>

Reward yourself for every successful task completed, no matter how small! Be your own cheerleader. Do something that will make you smile.

For suggestions on building your memory skills, refer to Chapter 15, Rebuilding Skills.

For more help with memory problems consult a speech and language therapist.

Keep in mind that some medications may interfere with memory. Check with your doctor to determine if any of the medications you are taking may cause memory loss as a side effect.

Medical History Form   Updated _____

Name _____
DOB _____
SS# _____
Address _____

_____

_____

Phone _____
Phone _____

Emergency Contact:
Name _____
Relationship _____
Phone _____
Phone _____

Allergies: _____

_____

_____

_____

Current Medications: _____

_____

_____

_____

_____

_____

_____

_____

**Supplements and
Over the Counter Medications:**

_____

_____

_____

_____

_____

Treating Physicians:

DR. _____
Specialty _____
Address _____

_____

Phone _____

DR. _____
Specialty _____
Address _____

_____

Phone _____

DR. _____
Specialty _____
Address _____

_____

Phone _____

DR. _____
Specialty _____
Address _____

_____

Phone _____

DR. _____
Specialty _____
Address _____

_____

Phone _____

Tools

Other Medications Tried and Reason Stopped: _____

_____

_____

_____

_____

_____

Surgeries and Injuries (include dates):

_____

_____

_____

_____

_____

_____

_____

Current Health Conditions:

_____

_____

_____

_____

_____

_____

_____

_____

_____

_____

Notes:_____

_____

_____

_____

_____

Family Health History:

Major Health Issues (Cause of Death)

Mother _____

Father _____

Siblings:

_____

_____

_____

_____

_____

_____

_____

Paternal Grandparents:

_____

_____

_____

Maternal Grandparents:

_____

_____

Tools

Frequently Dialed Phone Numbers

Keep it handy. Post near phone or keep in the back of your phonebook.

Tools

Family	Medical

Friends	Other

Telephone Log

Use diffent colored paper for different issues.

	A	B	C	D	E
1	Date	Phone Number	Where Calling	Talked To	Summary and Follow-Up Needed
2					
3					
4					
5					
6					
7					

Tools

Getting Out the Door Checklist
Post in the front of your planner or near the front door.

First: Check your notes in your Calendar or Planner

❏ _____

Second: Do you have everything you need?

❏ Keys
❏ Wallet/purse and money
❏ ID/Store discount card
❏ Lists - errands, grocery
❏ Planner
❏ Paperwork for meeting/appointments
❏ Items for errands – mail, banking
❏ Cell phone
❏ Directions
❏ Water bottle
❏ Glasses, sunglasses
❏ _____

Third: Before you leave the house:

❏ Turn off the stove, iron
❏ Turn off the lights, computer
❏ Turn down the heat
❏ Take out the dog, bring in the cat
❏ Lock the back door
❏ _____

NOTES:

It is very helpful to prepare paperwork for appointments the day before.

Consider leaving a spare key with a family member, a trusted friend or neighbor or hidden in a secure place, to prevent panic if you accidentally lock yourself out of the house or car.

Memory Jogger List

To Create "To Do" List (Remember to check your calendar or planner as well.)

Home

- ❑ Phone calls
- ❑ Mail
- ❑ Computer
- ❑ Organize
- ❑ Laundry
- ❑ Clean
- ❑ Cook
- ❑ Yard work
- ❑ Home projects
- ❑ Other: _____

Errands

- ❑ Bank
- ❑ Grocery store
- ❑ Pharmacy
- ❑ Gas
- ❑ Haircut
- ❑ Greeting cards, gifts
- ❑ Movie rentals
- ❑ Other: _____

Medical

- ❑ Appointments
- ❑ Insurance
- ❑ Other: _____

Financial

- ❑ Bills
- ❑ Bank statement
- ❑ Taxes
- ❑ Other: _____

Legal

- ❑ _____
- ❑ _____

Friends/Social

- ❑ Email
- ❑ Birthdays
- ❑ Notes - thank yous, sympathy
- ❑ Meeting friends
- ❑ Family outings
- ❑ Holidays
- ❑ Other: _____

Pets

- ❑ _____
- ❑ _____

Special Occasions

- ❑ Social events – parties, weddings, sporting events
- ❑ Children's plays, ceremonies,
- ❑ Company
- ❑ Other: _____

Projects:

- ❑ _____
- ❑ _____
- ❑ _____
- ❑ _____
- ❑ _____
- ❑ _____
- ❑ _____
- ❑ _____

Tools

Memory Tips and Strategies

Medications

Pill boxes. Place pills where you'll see them when you need to take them. Cues on watch or phones.

Grooming appropriately

Checklist on mirror. Place toiletries in plain sight. Put them away as you use them.

Dressing appropriately

Lay out everything you are going to wear the night before on a designated hook or chair.

Things "To Do"

Lists. Prioritize. Place materials needed for the day on a table that is seldom used and put them away as tasks are accomplished.

Finding things at home – dishes, laundry, groceries

Put labels on the outside of drawers and cabinets. Keep similar items together and close to where you will use them.

Procedures for tasks like bill paying, computer

Memory jogger lists of steps, 5x7 cards. Color codes for different tasks.

Names

Make notes beside their names when in meetings or on the phone. Keep it in the folder for that issue. Review family photos before family gatherings.

Telephone Numbers and Addresses

Divide address book into categories – friends, family, medical, etc. Post lists of frequently used numbers near phones.

Telephone messages

Keep a notebook and pencil near each phone. Check √ when call is returned.

Why you called someone

Before you call - make a list.

Result of phone calls

Make notes right after a call. Keep a log for ongoing issues.

Remembering thoughts long enough to participate in conversations without interrupting

In meetings or on the phone, sit with paper and pencil in front of you.
Note a few key words to cue you. You can refer back to it at an appropriate time.
Let it be OK to do more listening.

Appointments

Ask for and save appointment cards to refer to. Keep ONE calendar, organizer, planner or appointment book. Use different colored inks or cues, like squares or circles, for different types of appointments and designating priorities.

Paperwork for appointments

Get ready 1-2 days before the appointment, including insurance issues and co-pays.

Questions for doctors

Designate a section of your organizer/planner and make a list as questions arise. Review before the appointment.

Instructions from appointments

Ask for an appointment card and a copy of instructions in writing that you can review later, when you are less stressed and not worrying if you wrote them correctly.

Car keys, eyeglasses, wallet/purse, phone

Keep everything together. Establish one designated place to keep them where you will see them when you're going out the door. You can also use checklists posted at the door.

Driving routes and directions

A day or two before, consult a map or computer directions and call for landmarks if possible. Be sure to get reverse directions for return trip as well! Program your GPS before you leave the house.

Where you parked the car

Try to park your car in the same area of the parking lot each time you go to that store. You can also make a written or voice note when you park.

Thoughts forgotten before you get home

Carry a mini-recorder or use the message feature on your phone. Keep a notebook and pen in your purse or pocket and in the car.

Ingredients when cooking

Place all ingredients on the counter and put them away as you finish with them. Use a pencil to make checkmarks on recipes. Use a very large measuring cup so you can see how much you have added.

When something is in the oven

Carry a timer with you or around your neck. Stay in the kitchen and work on something else, your nose may help remind you!

What you read

Start small – magazine articles, children's books. Reread, read out loud, take notes, summarize to yourself or to someone else.

Finding information you read

Removable page flags, pencil check marks, colored highlighters.

Following TV Programs

Use headphones to help screen out distractions. Record and watch again.

Typing

Re-teach yourself with a beginner's program for the computer.

Math

Re-teach yourself. Do it in pencil and check it with a calculator but don't rely on calculators totally. You won't re-learn it!

Hobbies you used to enjoy

Re-teach yourself. Get out the instruction books or get one at the library. Start with beginner's books, take an adult education class on it.

A Prosthesis for Your Memory

Strategies For Setting Up Organizers

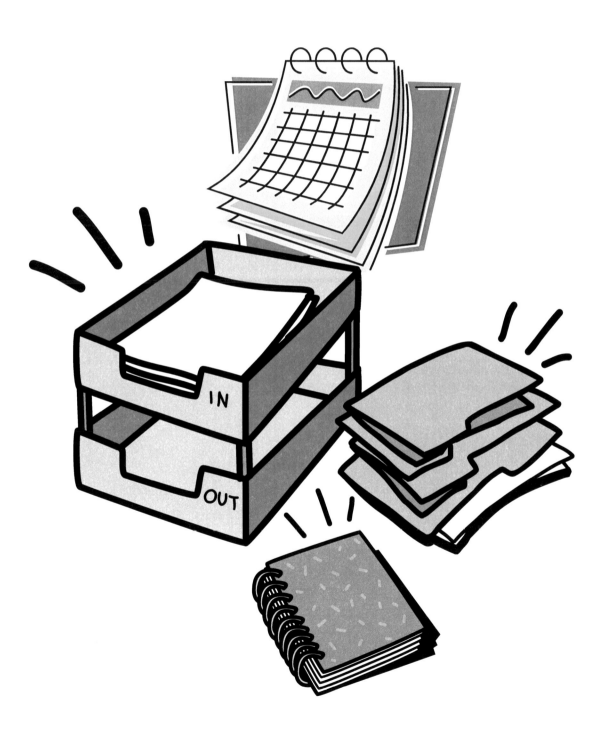

A Prosthesis for Your Memory

Strategies for Setting Up Organizers

"We are not retreating – we are advancing in another direction."

— Douglas MacArthur

A calendar, planner or organizer is like a "prosthesis" or substitute, for your memory. It is a method for keeping track of all the information you need to run your daily life effectively. Most survivors would be lost without one. Many people who don't have a brain injury use them to manage their busy lives. So try to think of using an organizer as a "strategy for success".

Suggestions for Setting Up an Organizer

Step 1

Identify the things that you need to keep track of:

- ❏ Appointments
- ❏ Things "to do"
- ❏ Daily schedule/time management
- ❏ Telephone numbers and addresses
- ❏ People's names
- ❏ Birthdays/anniversaries
- ❏ Cues for medication, etc.
- ❏ Questions for doctors
- ❏ Routes and maps
- ❏ Daily log or diary
- ❏ Procedures for tasks
- ❏ Goals, objectives and plans to achieve goals
- ❏ Expenses/bills
- ❏ Shopping lists/things to buy
- ❏ Project planning
- ❏ Car inspection and maintenance

_____

_____

_____

_____

Step 2

Decide what kind of organizer system fits the needs you have identified. Choose **ONE** planning system. For example: trying to use a calendar and a weekly planner to keep track of appointments can be confusing. You end up with multiple places to record information and keep information current. You soon lose track of which is accurate.

Systems to consider

- ❏ Weekly planner/organizer (purchased where office supplies are sold)
- ❏ Three ring notebooks with dividers
- ❏ Wall calendar
- ❏ Small pocket calendar
- ❏ Large dry erase board
- ❏ Home computer
- ❏ Portable electronic organizer

Step 3

Choose the format that best suits your needs, some considerations:

- ❏ A larger format is easier to read and write in.
- ❏ A smaller format will be more convenient to carry, consider mobility issues.
- ❏ A week-at-a-glance will allow you to plan your energy.
- ❏ An electronic organizer is expensive and requires learning.
- ❏ A computer or wall calendar may allow you to track activities for multiple people in the family.

Step 4

Begin using your organizer for the most important things you need to keep track of first - probably appointments, your daily schedule and your To Do List.

Resist duplicating organizing systems.

For example, keeping track of appointments on a wall calendar at home *and* in your daily planner or electronic organizer means you have two places to add information and make changes. It is more work and almost always becomes confusing.

Sometimes it makes sense to use a different system for a specific task.

You can have an address book at home for friends and family and an address section in your planner for medical contacts so you have them with you when you are out of the house.

Don't eliminate any system you already have in place if it is working for you.

For example, if you use a wall calendar at home to keep track of appointments and it works well for you, continue to use that system.

Suggestions for Using a Planning Tool Effectively

<u>Step 1</u>

Schedule in all appointments and commitments first.

Schedule in at least **double** travel time. Allow time from door to door, including extra time for:

- ❏ Traffic
- ❏ Wrong turns
- ❏ Finding parking
- ❏ Waiting for the elevator
- ❏ Finding the office
- ❏ Using the restroom
- ❏ Registering
- ❏ Time to collect yourself before the appointment

This one strategy will greatly reduce your stress and help you arrive relaxed and focused and able to accomplish what you need to.

<u>Step 2</u>

Schedule "must dos" in "peak performance" time. At what time of day are you most alert and attentive?

Schedule activities that require less mental effort during periods in which you tend to be less alert and attentive.

<u>Step 3</u>

Schedule a midday/early afternoon "down time" - a "brain recharging break" or a nap as a "performance strategy"!

<u>Step 4</u>

Schedule *daily* planning time, 30-60 minutes, usually first thing in the morning. If you have an early morning appointment, it might be helpful to plan to do this the night before. Planning time tasks:

1. Put away any paperwork from the previous day that is in your planner, folder or notebook.
2. Transfer any undone tasks from the day before.
3. Review your tasks for the day and make sure you have any necessary paperwork ready for appointments.
4. Check off the tasks in your planner as you complete them. (You can make a box or line beside each task.)
5. Use colors to help cue you, like different colored inks for different activities – blue for appointments, black for To Do List, purple for birthdays, red arrows for priorities - use your favorite colors!

Step 5

Schedule *weekly* planning time – at the end or the beginning of each week - schedule time to review your To Do List and plan your tasks for the week. If you have a family, preview the week together.

Step 6

Schedule *monthly* planning time – at the end or the beginning of each month – schedule time to review your To Do List and plan your month, time to check your Master Bill List and organize the next month's bills and appointments.

Take your planner/organizer with you wherever you go.

The more frequently you refer to the information, the more familiar and easier it will become.

If you choose a system that you don't carry with you to your appointments, then you need another system for entering information and keeping it up to date.

For example, if you use a computer or wall calendar as your main planning tool, you can take a folder to appointments. When you get home from the appointment, place the folder on your desk where you will see it to remind you to take care of any follow up.

Use your planner to help you realistically set limits on your time and energy.

Consult it before you say "yes" and regret it. Use your planner:

❏ When scheduling appointments

❏ When someone asks you to do something that you aren't sure you will be able to do. Develop the habit of saying, "'Let me check my calendar first."

Computers and electronic organizers can be helpful planning tools.

They are especially helpful if you have difficulty writing. However, there are advantages and disadvantages to using electronic organizers to consider.
See "Cell Phones and Electronic Organizers" following this section.

Save your calendars from year to year.

They can provide irreplaceable memory cues if you need to fill out review forms for insurance or Social Security.

Cell Phones and Electronic Organizers

Today's cell phones and electronic organizers are amazing little multi-tasking tools, allowing you to record, store and access unlimited information as well as be constantly connected to others. They are loaded with multiple applications that can be easily identified by picture icons and opened with the brush of a fingertip. Some have software that makes them easier for people with disabilities to use, like voice message recording or speech to text. However, as they become more complex, they can also become more challenging for people with brain injury to learn and use. Cell phones and electronic organizers have many of the same functions these days. You may find all the functions you need on your cell phone. Below are some practical suggestions to consider, no matter which electronic device you choose.

Suggestions

Keep it as simple as possible.

Think about what functions or applications will help you the most and start with just those few functions. The phone, appointment/medication reminders and voice recording functions are commonly most helpful for survivors.

Consider having unused functions deactivated or blocked.

This helps you avoid unwanted expenses.

Learn one function at time.

Figure out what function is most important to you and use your electronic device for just that single purpose until you feel you have mastered it. Then move on to learning the next function.

Develop a system of checking it and updating it.

Do this just like you would with a calendar or weekly planner system. For example, every Sunday evening you might check for appointments and reminders and log in new information.

This is the biggest key to success when using any organization system, remembering to use it, to check it and keep it current!

Back up, back up, back up information stored in your electronic devices.

It's wonderful to have all that information at your fingertips but it won't be so wonderful to have it disappear in a flash if your device is damaged, lost or stolen. Some devices allow you to merge your information with your computer, just be sure to do it on a regular basis.

Save your calendars.

They can provide irreplaceable memory cues later if you need to provide information to your insurance company or Social Security Disability regarding your doctor appointments or daily activities.

Manage your electronic device, don't let it manage you!

If you let it, your electronic device can run your life – constantly ringing, interrupting you anywhere, any time. Let it be ok, not to have it on all the time. Trying to answer it anytime, anywhere will disrupt your focus, concentration and memory - so how much will it really help you in the long run?

Don't let your cell phone/electronic organizer cause you to be disruptive or rude.

Avoid using it while you are in a meeting or at a function, even if you are just checking your email or texting and not talking out loud. You are dividing your attention and decreasing your cognition. Also, think about how you would feel if you were talking to someone or speaking to a group and your audience was focused on an electronic device instead of you.

Pull over to a safe place before using any electronic device when you are driving!

It can be very tempting to answer that ringtone but it is also extremely dangerous. Keep your phone out of reach, in the glove compartment or on the back seat if you have to. Better yet, turn it off while you are driving.
Know the laws pertaining to cell phone use and driving in your state.

Some features to consider before purchasing an electronic device:

- ❏ Safety, being able to contact someone in case of emergency, anywhere, anytime. This can literally be a lifesaver!
- ❏ Communication, anywhere, anytime. You don't need to be home to make and answer calls.
- ❏ Compact and easy to carry with you.
- ❏ Portable reminders for medications and appointments. Very handy!
- ❏ Internal phone book, eliminating the need to remember phone numbers or carry them with you separately.
- ❏ Voice messaging, easy to make reminders to yourself when away from home or when not convenient to write it down.
- ❏ Ability to check your calendar and make changes when away from home, if you choose to use that feature.
- ❏ Tool to keep track of money spent or debit card transactions.
- ❏ Easy access to huge amounts of information at your fingertips if you choose to have access to your email and/or the Internet.
- ❏ Options for larger screens and keyboards for ease of use.
- ❏ Ability to change background color and brightness on the screen, especially if you have vision problems.
- ❏ Multiple features on one device; can be helpful, can be confusing.
- ❏ You may want a cell phone that is just a cell phone.
- ❏ Long battery life is important – ask about it.
- ❏ Expense: a basic model may be the best fit for you and save you some money.
- ❏ A manual that is easy to understand.

If you grew up hearing, "Don't play with it, you'll break it," try to forget it. Playing with it is how you learn to use these devices.

Can you line up some technical support while you are learning your device, a patient friend or family member that you can consult regularly until you are familiar with your device? This will be extremely helpful.

Keep it simple and resist the urge to feel that you need to use a particular electronic device just because it seems everyone else does. You need to decide what is best for you and your circumstances.

"You may fail at what you do but you cannot fail at who you are."

— Unknown

Remember that in the big picture of life, your **To Do List** is not as important as your **To BE List.** Schedule time to be with the people you love and to do the things you love to do. It will help prevent fatigue, meltdowns, shutdowns and burn out.

Know that all of this tedious planning and organizing will get easier with practice. You will figure out how to plan your days and weeks to give you the balance you need.

For more help setting up organizers, consult an occupational therapist or a speech and language therapist.

64

Creating Shortcuts for Your Memory

Strategies for Getting Organized and Staying That Way!

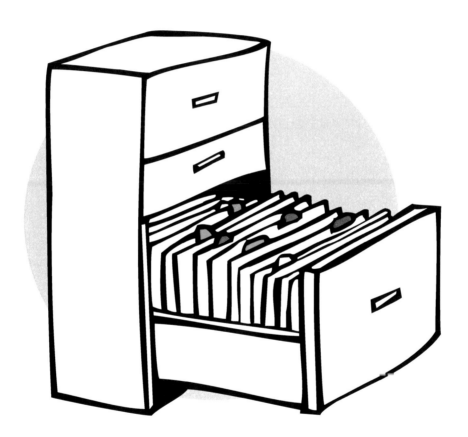

Creating Shortcuts for Your Memory

Strategies for Getting Organized and Staying That Way!

"When one door closes, another one opens ... but it is hell in the hallway."

— Man who lost his job and changed careers

Organizing really isn't that complicated, you already do it! Organizing is putting cards of the same suit together when you play cards, putting all the canned goods in the same cabinet in your kitchen or putting all the documents on one topic in a folder on your computer. Organizing is basically "putting like things together". When you are organized, you don't have to go through a lot of cards, cabinets, files or piles to find something. You know where to look. Working in an organized manner creates shortcuts for your memory!

Organizing and planning can help you think things through, stay focused and minimize getting surprised or feeling "ambushed" by something you didn't expect. When you plan your trip to the grocery store and organize a shopping list, you are much more likely to come home with what you need! Organization is a key "strategy for success".

Three Basic Tips for Successful Organizing

Tip #1 Avoid Reorganizing

Don't reorganize anything you already have a system for, whether it is clothes in your closet, your kitchen, or your files. Instead, build on the systems you already have, adding labels, colors, see-through containers, etc.

It is easier to relearn a system that has already been established than it is to start over and learn a new system.

Tip #2 Get Organized

1. **Think categories** - like rooms in a house.

   What items belong in the bathroom? What items belong in the kitchen?

   What belongs in my insurance file?

2. **Put "like things" together.** For example:
   - ❏ Group all your shirts together in your closet.
   - ❏ Group all the soups together in the kitchen.
   - ❏ Group all toiletries together in the bathroom or linen closet.
   - ❏ Group all the paperwork on an issue in one file or folder.

3. **Choose a location** for each group of items and try to put things back in their established places - *always!*

Tip #3 Stay Organized

This means putting things back where they came from or where they belong. I know, I sound like your mother - but this is probably the most important tip. It will save you a lot of energy, clutter, frustration and re-organizing in the long run!

Set aside time to do this daily. Get your children involved. I do this after I finish a project and before I start preparing supper, every day.

General Organizing Strategies

<u>Establish days for regular weekly activities and chores.</u>

Example:

> Sunday = refill pillbox and check prescriptions for refills needed
> Monday = paperwork and planning day
> Tuesday = errands
> Wednesday = grocery shopping day
> Thursday = laundry
> Friday = time for self!
> Saturday = family/friends day

<u>Collect the items you need to take with you when you leave the house that day.</u>

Put them beside something you always take when you leave the house, like your wallet and keys. For example:

- ❏ Before going grocery shopping: place every thing you need to take with you next to your wallet and keys to help you remember to take the items with you when you leave the house.

- ❏ Before a medical appointment: gather all the paperwork you will need for the appointment and put it in your planner or a folder. Place it next to your wallet and keys to help you remember to take it with you to the appointment.

<u>Organize work areas.</u>

Keep all the items you need to do something close to each other or place them all in the same area before you start. It will be easier to stay focused and complete the job if you don't have to move from area to area or hunt for supplies. For example:

- ❏ Put your bills to pay, calculator, envelopes, stamps and file for paid bills close to the area where you pay your bills.

- ❏ Store everything you use to change the oil in your car in one location.

- ❏ Pull out all the ingredients for a recipe before you begin.

- ❏ Get out everything you need to do gardening or yard work before you start.

<u>Think where would I look for this? (think categories)</u>

That's where you put it away. Put similar items together.

<u>Decide what goes where.</u>

You can use the "Hot/Warm/Cool Rule". The more frequently something is used, the warmer it is. Keep "hot" items, items that are used daily, easily accessible. Store them at waist height as much as possible. Items that you rarely use can be stored in less accessible places like the back of closets, attic or basement. The kitchen is a really good place to use this strategy.

<u>Establish a place to lay out **all** the items you are going to wear in the morning.</u>

Designate a special hook or chair. This habit is especially helpful before early morning appointments or special occasions.

Strategies for Organizing Paperwork

<u>When organizing "To Do Lists"</u>

❏ Think categories:

> Home chores, calls to make, things to buy, etc.
> (See Memory Jogger List in Chapter 4 on Memory.)

❏ Prioritize your lists into three sections:

- ○ "Must Dos" – usually time sensitive
- ○ Necessary to do
- ○ Would be nice to do if time

❏ Divide lists into manageable chunks of just 2-3 steps. It is easier to think through, less overwhelming.

❏ Make a line or box to check when a task is completed.

❏ Arrange errand and shopping lists to minimize backtracking and driving time, to save time and energy. If there are any "Must Dos" on your list, start there. Otherwise, start with the store farthest away from home. Then if you get overtired and aren't able to complete your list, you will be closer to home. Consult a map if you are unsure. If you are going to a mall, you can use one of their maps to plan and save yourself steps.

❏ Schedule breaks. Plan time to rest and have a snack, to recharge.

❏ Create scripts when needed. These are sublists of steps telling you when and what to do. They help you remember the details that go with a complex task like getting ready to go on vacation.
(See the Travel Checklist at end of this chapter.)

❏ Make multiple copies of frequently used lists or laminate a master copy. Try using different colors for different tasks or index cards for each step.

<u>Using folders</u>

❏ Use different colored folders to keep track of information for each category. For example, you can use a red folder for insurance papers, a blue folder for medical questions and instructions, a green folder for financial issues, different colors for each child's school info, etc. Use whatever colors make sense to you.

❏ Keep copies of all relevant paperwork in the corresponding folder.

❏ Keep a Telephone Log in the front of each folder. (See sample in Chapter 4 on Improving Memory.)

❏ Take the corresponding folder with you to your appointments.

❏ If you have trouble carrying folders or if the information tends to slip out, try pocket folders, a notebook with a zippered cover, a backpack or some kind of a bag or briefcase.

❏ Keep folders for active issues where you can see them. This creates a visual cue for yourself. You can use a separate pile on your desk topped with a decorative paperweight, a colorful milk crate or file cabinet close to your desk. Another system is the three-basket system for Incoming, Active and To Be Filed.

❏ If you have trouble remembering where to file something, try standing a ruler in its place when you pull it out to work on, like a bookmark. Then you will know right where it goes when you are ready to file it. Rulers are very inexpensive.

Traveling

1. <u>Create a master packing list:</u> (sample at end of chapter)

    ❏ Remember things that help you with your injuries like medications, your cap, earplugs, sunglasses, relaxation tapes, heating pad and ice pack.

    ❏ You can make copies of your master list for future trips or you can put it in a sheet saver and use a dry erase marker to check things off.

    ❏ Keep the list in your suitcase for future trips.

2. <u>Make a travel checklist</u> (sample at end of chapter)

    ❏ Use this to help you prepare and finish tasks you need to do before you leave. This might include ordering prescriptions, stopping the mail and making arrangements for pets.

    ❏ You can make copies for future trips or your can put it in a sheet saver and use a dry erase marker to check things off.

    ❏ Keep it in your suitcase for other trips.

3. <u>Navigating airports</u>

    ❏ You can find a map of most airports online. Print it out for each airport you will be in and carry it with you. This can be especially helpful when you are pressed for time.

There is no single "right way" to organize.
Experiment and find what works for you!

I think the only way to stay organized is to make yourself spend some time at it every day; putting things away, preventing clutter, helping your brain know where to find things. It gets easier once you establish places for things and have the routine for keeping up with it.

Get involved in art therapy or an art class if you can. Amazingly, working in any kind of art medium can help the brain reorganize!

For more help with organization, consult an occupational therapist or a speech and language pathologist. If insurance and finances allow, consider returning to therapy once a year to help you continue to progress.

Getting Organized Worksheet

Step 1

Check the areas where information is breaking down and you need to get more organized:

- ❏ Running out of medications
- ❏ Missing appointments
- ❏ Can't find information when needed
- ❏ Can't remember things or remember them incorrectly
- ❏ Can't remember personal information
- ❏ Losing things
- ❏ Not paying bills
- ❏ Getting lost
- ❏ Arriving late
- ❏ Leaving the house without things needed
- ❏ Arriving at appointments without information needed
- ❏ Leaving the house without brushing teeth or shaving, etc.
- ❏ Runnng out of food, clean laundry, medications, etc.
- ❏ Falling apart during the day
- ❏ Not preparing meals
- ❏ Planning for longer-term activities
- ❏ Other problem areas:

_____

_____

_____

_____

_____

Step 2

Start with the area that is causing you the most stress. Then list some ideas to improve your system. As you read future chapters you can add suggestions.

> Sample Challenge: Cook supper without falling apart.
>
> Strategies to try:
> - ✓ Take a rest break before starting to cook.
> - ✓ Start early, allow extra time.
> - ✓ Let the answering machine answer the phone.
> - ✓ Set the table and make the salad before starting to cook.

1. Challenge: _____

   Strategies to try:

   _____

   _____

   _____

   _____

   _____

2. Challenge: _____

   Strategies to try:

   _____

   _____

   _____

   _____

   _____

Notes:

Work on one challenge at a time. When you feel like that area is running smoother, go on to the next challenge. It can take several months to incorporate a new way of doing things before it becomes routine.

Acknowledge all improvements, no matter how small! Write them in your journal, share them with another survivor

Reverse Scheduling!

If you have trouble getting to appointments on time, try this! It looks complicated but follow the steps. After you do it a couple times, it will get a lot easier!

1. Sit down the day before your appointment and on a separate lined piece of paper, list everything you have to do before your meeting. Work in pencil, write the tasks in the order you do them.

   Example:

_____	Wake-up
_____	Shower
_____	Dress and groom (teeth, hair)
_____	Prepare and eat breakfast
_____	Let the dog out
_____	Check e-mail
_____	Check calendar/planner
_____	Check exit checklist and load car
_____	Do errands (get gas, bank)
_____	Travel time

2. Estimate how long each task will take.
   Example:

   15 min/ wake up

   15 min/ shower

   30 min/ dressing and grooming

   _____ / prepare and eat breakfast

   _____ / let the dog out

   _____ / check e-mail

   _____ / check calendar/planner

   _____ / check exit checklist and load car

   _____ / errands

   _____ / travel time

Tips:

Figure in *realistic* travel time; always allow extra time, for traffic, weather, parking, finding the office, etc.

When in doubt, allow extra time. You will think more clearly when you aren't stressed from rushing.

3. Write in your appointment time last, at the bottom of your list.

   Next, working from the bottom of the page to the top, make your timetable. Example:

_____	(15 min)	Wake-up
_____	(15 min)	Shower
_____	(30 min)	Dress and groom
_____	(20 min)	Prepare and eat breakfast
_____	(5 min)	Let the dog out
_____	(30 min)	Check e-mail
_____	(10 min)	Check planner/calendar
9:45		**DEPARTURE TIME**
9:45 –10:00	(15 min)	Check exit checklist and load car
3. 10:00 –10:30	(30 min)	Errands
2. 10:30-11:00	(30 min)	Travel time
1. **11:00**		**APPOINTMENT**

Now you have a strategy or plan for successfully arriving on time!

Additional Strategies:

Departure time

Set an alarm! You may have to make adjustments to your schedule if you become involved in a phone conversation or get sidetracked but if you can stick to the designated departure time, you will still be on track for success – arriving on time for your appointment!

The day before

Be sure to gather everything you need to take with you to the appointment, insurance forms, questions for the doctor. Put these items near your wallet and keys, where you will see them when you go out the door.

The night before

Consider what is appropriate to wear for your appointment in the morning and lay out <u>all</u> the items you are going to put on. This is a huge time saver, especially for early morning appointments. If it is a special occasion, you might even want to try everything on ahead of time, like a dress rehearsal.

After going through this process a few times, you will figure out where your timing problems are and you will become more efficient. You will figure out how much time you usually need to get up and out the door and you won't have to stop and figure it out step by step every time. It will get easier with practice!

Reward yourself for every appointment you arrive at on time, relaxed and with everything you need! Note how you feel! Take some time to do something that makes you smile. Perhaps you would like to stop for an ice cream or visit a friend on the way home!

Note:

This process is similar to how you plan preparation time for meals. Mealtime is your "appointment time". Starting with the dish that takes the longest to prepare, you work backwards to figure out necessary preparation and cooking time. Then you know when you need to begin! See Chapter 10 for more help with meal planning.

Tools

Packing List

Customize to suit your needs. Keep a copy in your suitcase.

Clothes

- ❏ Shirts and blouses
- ❏ Pants and shorts
- ❏ Dress, skirt
- ❏ Suit, suit jacket
- ❏ Coat, jacket
- ❏ Shoes, boots
- ❏ Underwear
- ❏ Bathing suit, hat
- ❏ Nylons
- ❏ _____
- ❏ _____
- ❏ _____
- ❏ _____
- ❏ _____

Toiletries

- ❏ Medications?
  Need refills, pack in carry-on
- ❏ Comb, brush
- ❏ Toothbrush and toothpaste
- ❏ Deodorant
- ❏ Razor and shaving cream
- ❏ Hair dryer, electric rollers
- ❏ Makeup
- ❏ Sunscreen
- ❏ Jewelry
- ❏ _____
- ❏ _____
- ❏ _____
- ❏ _____
- ❏ _____

Comfort Items

- ❏ Ear plugs, sunglasses, cap
- ❏ Relaxation music
- ❏ Heating pad, ice pack
- ❏ First aid items
- ❏ _____
- ❏ _____
- ❏ _____
- ❏ _____

Other

- ❏ Purse/wallet
- ❏ Keys – for return
- ❏ Cell phone and charger,
  pack in carry on
- ❏ Lap top and power cord
- ❏ Tickets, motel and rental car
  reservation information
- ❏ Maps/directions/tour books
- ❏ Necessary phone numbers
- ❏ Camera, batteries, charger
- ❏ Gift (for special occasions)
- ❏ Athletic equipment
- ❏ Car seat
- ❏ Activities for kids
- ❏ Books, magazines, snacks

Special Equipment/Materials

- ❏ _____
- ❏ _____
- ❏ _____
- ❏ _____
- ❏ _____

Tools

Travel Planning Script

Advance Preparations

Location and dates of travel: _____

Car Travel

- ❏ Maps/directions/tour books
- ❏ Check tires, fluids, belts
- ❏ Gas
- ❏ Pet carrier, water, food, leash, vaccination papers
- ❏ _____
- ❏ _____
- ❏ _____

Plane Travel

- ❏ Airline carrier _____
  Phone _____
- ❏ Travel agent _____
  Phone _____
- ❏ Shuttle service _____
  Phone _____
- ❏ Tickets
- ❏ Photo I.D.
- ❏ Seat assignments
- ❏ Map of airport from website
- ❏ _____
- ❏ _____

Bus/Train Travel

- ❏ Carrier _____
- ❏ Phone _____
- ❏ Tickets _____
- ❏ Schedule _____
- ❏ _____
- ❏ _____

Hotel

- ❏ Name of hotel _____
  Phone _____
- ❏ Reservation # _____
- ❏ Discount coupons/cards

Car Rental

- ❏ Car agency _____
  Phone _____
- ❏ Reservation # _____
- ❏ Discount coupons
- ❏ _____
- ❏ _____

Leaving Country

- ❏ Passport and photocopy – (pack copy separately)
- ❏ Visa
- ❏ Foreign currency
- ❏ Special medical arrangements
- ❏ Electrical converters
- ❏ _____
- ❏ _____

Other

- ❏ _____
- ❏ _____
- ❏ _____
- ❏ _____
- ❏ _____
- ❏ _____

Tools

Preparations Before Leaving

Medication Refills Needed

- ❏ _____
- ❏ _____
- ❏ _____
- ❏ _____

Pet Arrangements

- ❏ Kennel _____
  Phone _____

Bills Paid

- ❏ _____
- ❏ _____
- ❏ _____
- ❏ _____

Reschedule Appointments/ Services

- ❏ Notify school
- ❏ Notify regular sitter
- ❏ Notify lessons/activities
- ❏ Mail arrangements
- ❏ Stop newspaper(s)
- ❏ Ask neighbor to:
  Keep an eye on the house,
  collect unexpected packages,
  water plants, water garden
- ❏ _____
- ❏ _____
- ❏ _____
- ❏ _____
- ❏ _____
- ❏ _____
- ❏ _____

Inform Where You Can Be Reached

- ❏ _____
  Phone _____
- ❏ _____
  Phone _____
- ❏ _____
  Phone _____
- ❏ _____
  Phone _____

Other

- ❏ _____
- ❏ _____
- ❏ _____
- ❏ _____
- ❏ _____
- ❏ _____

Tools

Exit Checklist   <u>Before you leave the house</u>

Essentials

- ❏ Make sure you have your tickets!
- ❏ Check departure time for plane/train/bus
- ❏ Suitcases – final check of packing list

Carry-on Bags

- ❏ Remove forbidden items if traveling by plane (check website for restrictions)
- ❏ Medications – in case of delays

Purse/Wallet

- ❏ If traveling by plane, remove forbidden items
- ❏ Pack keys for return
- ❏ Credit card - remove unneeded credit cards
- ❏ Take health insurance card
- ❏ Cash needed for trip
- ❏ Traveler's checks – keep a separate record of check #s

Close Up House

- ❏ Empty perishables from refrigerator
- ❏ Run disposal, dishwasher
- ❏ Take out trash
- ❏ Water plants
- ❏ Shut off water for washer
- ❏ Unplug computers and TVs – in case of electrical storm
- ❏ Turn off/unplug where possible: stove and kitchen appliances
- ❏ Turn down thermostat
- ❏ Close and lock all windows
- ❏ Pull down shades/close drapes
- ❏ Set timers/leave a couple of lights on

Finally...

- ❏ Use bathroom
- ❏ Lock all doors
- ❏ Set alarm

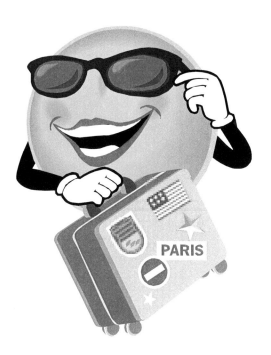

Tools

Steps To Success Example

Step 1   Project, issue, problem

Getting to doctor appointments on time

Step 2   What strategies might work? Have you been in a similar situation?

Prepare questions and co-pay ahead of time

Take copy of medical history

Take dry run to new location

Take appointment card with me

Allow extra travel time

Step 3   Picture the end goal. What would success look like?

Arriving at appointment on time and relaxed, having any paperwork prepared ahead of time and remembering to ask the doctor my questions.

Celebrating with ice cream on the way home!

Step 4   Outline your strategies, your steps – to Success!

Weekend before: Check directions and take dry run if necessary

Two days ahead: Gather copy of medical history, co-pay and list of questions for doctor

Night before: Lay out clothes to wear

Take calendar/planner and appointment card

Allow extra travel time

Step 5   Evaluation

What strategies worked?

All planning above

What didn't work?

Left the house late, forgot paperwork, got nervous, made a wrong turn and was late for appointment

Step 6   Suggestions for next time

Establish a "must leave the house time" and don't answer the phone while I am trying to get out the door.

Put everything I am going to need when I leave in the morning near my purse where I will see it and won't have to hunt for anything.

Steps To Success Worksheet

<u>Step 1</u>   Project, issue, problem

❏ _____
❏ _____
❏ _____

<u>Step 2</u>   What strategies might work? Have you been in a similar situation?

❏ _____
❏ _____
❏ _____
❏ _____
❏ _____

<u>Step 3</u>   Picture the end goal. What would success look like?

❏ _____
❏ _____
❏ _____

<u>Step 4</u>   Outline your strategies, your steps – to Success!

❏ _____
❏ _____
❏ _____
❏ _____
❏ _____

<u>Step 5</u>   Evaluation

What strategies worked?   What didn't work?

❏ _____   ❏ _____
❏ _____   ❏ _____
❏ _____   ❏ _____
❏ _____   ❏ _____

<u>Step 6</u>   Suggestions for next time

❏ _____
❏ _____
❏ _____

Tools

Turning a "Bad Brain Day" Into a "Good Brain Day"

Strategies for Improving Cognition

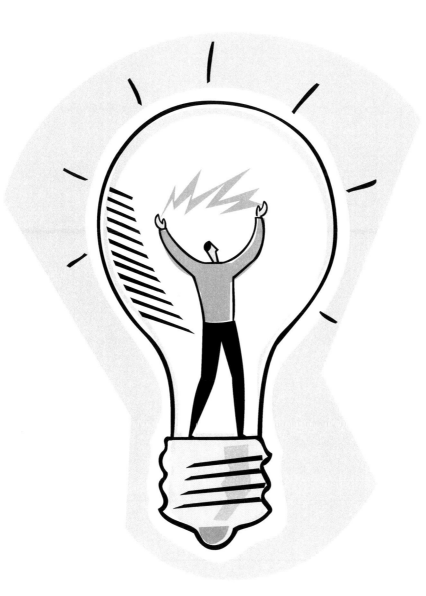

Turning a "Bad Brain Day" Into a "Good Brain Day"

Strategies for Improving Cognition

"The Recovery Journey is much like life itself ... Some things you can do, some things you can't, and a successful journey may often be made from discerning which is which. We survivors have to figure all that out not once, but twice."

— John Richards, Survivor

It can be difficult to measure progress when you are healing something you can't see, like your brain. If you get discouraged, look back at your journals or calendars. They will help you remember and realize just how far you have come.

Try working with things in different ways. We all have learning strengths and we take in information in multiple ways. (See the section "How Are You Smart?" at the end of this chapter.)

General Suggestions

Get a good night's sleep.

If you are not sleeping well, you won't be able to recharge and heal and you won't be able to think well. (See suggestions in Chapter 2.)

Consult your doctor if you think you might be depressed.

Depression inhibits cognition.

Do your best to maintain a healthy diet and drink plenty of water.

Your brain is one of the first organs to dehydrate.

Slow down!

Slowing down and doing things step by step in a quiet atmosphere will help you stay focused and remember what you did. Pushing, rushing, trying to do more than one thing at a time all create stress and inhibit cognition. I know, it feels counterproductive, but it isn't. Try it!

Determine your best time of day for learning.

Try to schedule challenging tasks when you are most alert, your "prime brain time". For some of us it is in the morning and for others it is in the evening.

<u>Set yourself up to succeed.</u>

Work in a "memory friendly" environment, minimize distractions and interruptions. This is the first and probably most important strategy my therapists taught me. It enabled me to start having success.

- ❏ Take the dog out before you begin.
- ❏ Get your cup of coffee/tea/water before you start.
- ❏ Let phone calls go to the answering machine and turn down the volume while you are working.
- ❏ Try to put your worries on hold for the time being.

Repetitions

Repetition is the foundation of the learning/rehabilitation process. Repetition creates a pattern, a pathway. Repetitions also give you an opportunity to note improvement with each repetition!

- ❏ Don't be afraid to ask for information and instructions to be repeated. Write them down if possible. Repeat back to check for accuracy.
- ❏ Use tape recorders, message machines and DVD recorders so you can replay and aid memory. Be sure to ask permission to record conversations.
- ❏ Take notes at meetings, when reading, on the telephone.
- ❏ Ask for information in writing or a summary of an important meeting when possible, especially regarding medical or legal information. Then you won't question the accuracy of what you wrote and you can reread it later when you are better able to focus.
- ❏ Take advantage of opportunities to repeat doing things.

    For example:
    - ○ Listening to phone messages as many times as needed
    - ○ Reading and rereading material
    - ○ Recording and watching your favorite television show more than once
    - ○ Watching a movie a second time, or a third.
    - ○ Attending the same workshops more than once
    - ○ Auditing a class before you take it
    - ○ Taking dry runs in the car to find a location before a meeting or appointment

Teach to learn.

Try teaching whatever you are working on to a child, a friend or family member. If no one is available, try reading your material aloud a few times.

<u>Trouble getting started (initiation)?</u>

Understanding why motivation and initiation can be such big problems after a brain injury can be helpful.

Common causes:

❏ Recollection of past problems, decisions, actions and successes may be impaired, limiting experiences to build upon.

❏ Cognitive fatigue may play a big role.

❏ The ability to self-regulate or self-monitor may be impaired.

❏ Activities may be overwhelming or too complex to deal with after an injury without breaking them down and developing strategies, making tasks even more complex in the beginning.

❏ To have motivation there must be a certain level of confidence, persistence and support. Motivation is based on hope, hope that you will succeed, based on past experiences of success. Survivors need to relearn everything and begin to question everything they do.

❏ Some medications can inhibit motivation. If you are having difficulties in this area, check with your doctor to make sure your medications aren't contributing to the problem.

Try these strategies:

❏ Plan a reward for when you complete the task!

❏ Think priorities - are there any deadlines to consider?

❏ Begin by pulling out all the materials you need for the task, like the ingredients for a recipe so they will be handy and you won't get sidetracked looking for something.

❏ Put on some uplifting instrumental music.

❏ Check your Memory Jogger List of categories and make a "To Do List". (See sample Memory Jogger List in Memory, chapter 4.)

❏ Break the job down into smaller chunks of 2-3 steps each.

❏ A 15-minute "brain warm-up", like working on a crossword, sudoku, or jigsaw puzzle.

❏ Take a short a walk, walk the dog, do some stretching exercises or a small physical chore to "wake up".

❏ Do some Brain Gym exercises if you are familiar with Brain Gym.

❏ Partner with someone who will coach you and give you gentle reminders.

<u>Trouble staying focused and on task?</u>

Try:

- ❑ Working in a clear space with only the materials you need for the task in your work area to minimize distractions.
- ❑ Working on one thing at a time, one step at a time. Avoid dividing your attention.
- ❑ Working at your own pace, don't rush.
- ❑ Using earplugs or headphones to shut out distractions. (Headphones will show others you are trying to concentrate.)
- ❑ Playing soft background music or using a fan or white noise machine.
- ❑ Chewing on a coffee stirrer or some strong flavored gum or candy.
- ❑ Using yellow tinted glasses to reduce the glare of bright or florescent lights.

<u>Do you feel "stuck" like there is a "logjam" in your brain?</u>

Try to figure out why. Are you hungry? Are you in pain? Are you feeling overwhelmed? Are you getting distracted? Are you getting tired?

- ❑ TAKE A BREAK! If it feels especially hard to take a break, it may be what you need to do the most. You are probably pushing too hard. The more difficult the task, the more breaks you will need.
- ❑ I know it isn't how you got things done before but believe me, it will help you to do more now. How much are you getting done being "stuck" anyway?
- ❑ Make sure you are working in good posture to minimize pain and fatigue.
- ❑ Switch to a physical task for a short while like putting away dishes or folding laundry.
- ❑ Put on some instrumental background music.
- ❑ Make a timetable for yourself; be sure to allow for pacing and breaks.
- ❑ Use cues, like an alarm on a watch or a computer, as reminders.
- ❑ Use a timer (digital or without a ticking sound to distract you).
- ❑ Can you tackle the task from a different direction, bringing in a visual or a "hands on" component? (See "How You Are Smart?" at the end of this chapter.)

<u>Sometimes two steps backward = one step forward.</u>

Keep in mind that you may need to get out the instructions for things you used to know how to do "automatically", like how to use an appliance, tools, camera, etc. You may need to go back and reteach yourself some skills. To relearn typing, you may need to get a beginner's typing tutorial. To relearn music, you may need to start with a beginner's music book.

Resist ruling out possibilities. The future may surprise you. Healing from a brain injury takes time, a long time. Sometimes you can relearn something at a much faster pace than when you learned it originally.

Pacing and Breaks

<u>Try alternating cognitive and physical activities.</u>

Do this throughout the day.

<u>Balance work and play.</u>

Be sure to include time to do little things that you enjoy doing each day. Pick things that make you smile or make it a "good day" for you like playing with a pet or talking to a friend. You will work more efficiently and you will feel better doing it.

<u>Watch for signs of stress.</u>

Stress interferes with cognition. Fatigue, increased pain, increasing mistakes, increased sensitivities to light or sound, feeling edgy or anxious or feeling "stuck", are all signs of stress and time to take a break. If a break doesn't help, it is time to stop.

Keep Challenging Yourself

"Challenging your brain creates new neural pathways. Just like you challenge a muscle to grow it, well, the brain gets new connections. Want to keep your brain young? Exercise it."

— Dr. Mehmet Oz,
You: The Owner's Manual

Even learning just a word, helps build mental bridges that link information and make it easier to retrieve. Accomplishments build self-confidence. "Self-confidence is the number-one memory builder."

— Dennis P. Swiercinsky,
50 Ways You Can Improve Your Memory

Think Progress

Start your day with the question:
What would be a good sign of progress for me today?
End your day with the question:
What little bit of progress did I make today?
What little bit of progress would I like to achieve tomorrow?
Keep a Victory Log and write a journal marking progress and goals met.

— D. Bissonnette,
30 Ways to Shine

Strive to think *how* can I turn this into a "good brain day"?

Try not to think about the need to use all these strategies in negative terms, think of it as a "Strategy for Success"!

Reward yourself for every successful task completed, no matter how small!

Pat yourself on the back. We have to be our own cheerleaders now.

Some days just won't be "good brain days". Some days you know you will just end up making mistakes and being frustrated. Some days it is actually more productive to surrender, acknowledge reality and do something less taxing or better yet, recharging.

For more help in these areas contact a Speech and Language Pathologist. They can help not only with problems concerning written and spoken language but also difficulties with memory, processing and organization.

Some medications can interfere with cognition. Check with your doctor to determine if any of the medications you are taking may cause memory loss as a side effect.

How Are You Smart?!

Answer each question by checking the box on the left that best describes how you usually work best. Ignore the list on the right for now.

How do you like to figure things out that come with instructions?

❏ Have someone explain it to you?   Auditory

❏ Have someone show you how to do it?   Visual

❏ Read the instructions first?   Visual

❏ Look at the pictures first?   Visual

❏ Dig right in, putting it together with your hands? Hands-on

When someone gives you driving directions, do you remember them best by:

❏ Hearing them?   Auditory

❏ Looking for landmarks?   Visual

❏ Writing them down?   Visual/Hands-on

❏ Taking a "dry run" in the car?   Hands-on

When you recall an event or situation, do you remember most:

❏ What was said?   Auditory

❏ Where you were?   Visual

❏ What you did?   Hands-on

Do your thoughts come more easily:

❏ When you hear someone talk about something?   Auditory

❏ When you look at pictures about it?   Visual

❏ When you write about it?   Hands-on

Now go back and circle the word on the right that corresponds to each of the boxes you checked on the left.

Are you a stronger auditory, visual or hands-on learner? _____

Your learning style can change with a brain injury. Generally we are trained and expected to process huge amounts of information auditorily - to hear it and know it. After a brain injury, we often don't process auditory information as well.
No wonder we have problems!

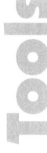

If you are more of a visual learner you may be helped by:

❑ Using colors and labels for files and organizing.

❑ Using clear containers in closets and the refrigerator so you can see the contents.

❑ Referring to photos and diagrams for instructions.

❑ Noting landmarks, signs and maps with directions.

❑ Laying out all materials for a project or ingredients for a recipe before you begin.

❑ Having someone *show* you how to do something, rather than explain it or read about it.

If you are more of a hands-on learner you may be helped by:

❑ Digging right in and physically working with something with your hands, rather than reading the instructions or having someone tell you how to do it.

❑ Doing dry runs in the car for learning directions.

❑ Laying files out on a table or the floor and moving them around to organize them.

❑ Taking notes.

❑ Having someone coach you while you try to do something, rather than show you while you watch or just tell you the instructions.

❑ Chewing on a plastic coffee stirrer, sucking on hard candy, or drinking something when you try to concentrate.

❑ Sitting on a therapy ball at the table so you can move around while you work.

We all have learning strengths

We take in information in many ways. Try working with materials in different ways. Once you discover your learning style and what strategies are most helpful, you can carry them over from task to task. Successive tasks will get easier!

"There is genius in all of us."

— Albert Einstein

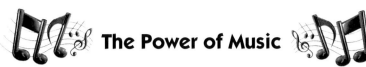 The Power of Music

Have you tried music therapy? Music is the tool I use the most to help me concentrate and focus, as well as to relax. It works so well for me, I was inspired to do some research. Music therapy is actually an ancient tradition, used in cultures throughout the world. Spiritual healers have used drums, bells and rattles to drive out disease, depression and despair since the dawn of humanity.

You've heard Musak Corporation's designer music in elevators, offices and stores. Music in the workplace has been shown to raise performance levels, productivity and sales significantly.

You've probably heard about the studies that show how soothing sounds can have amazing healing effects; lower the stress hormone cortisol, boost endorphins and IgA disease-fighting antibodies, reduce pain and lower blood pressure. Thirty minutes of classical music produced the same effect as 10mg. of Valium in a study at St. Agnes Hospital in Baltimore, MD!

Have you heard of "The Mozart Effect" – stimulating memory, intellectual and creative development with the music of Mozart? According to Don Campbell, author of *The Mozart Effect* and educator on the connection between music and healing, students who sing or play an instrument scored up to 51 points higher on SATs than the national average. He advocates listening to Mozart's unique music for just twenty minutes to:

♪ Increase concentration and memory

♪ Inspire right brain creative processing

♪ Increase spatial intelligence and change perception of time

♪ Enhance mood, motivation and pacing

♪ Improve body movement and coordination

As music therapy director Concetta Tomaino explains, memory seems to be preserved but it cannot always be retrieved. Music holds a key to gaining access to the system of memory retrieval. Alzheimer and Parkinson's patients who have lost their inner bearings often respond to music when all else has failed. When the brain is damaged, music "builds a bridge" as Dr. Samuel Wong describes it.

According to Campbell, listening to music can help balance the more logical left and the more intuitive right hemispheres of the brain. This interplay is thought to be the basis of creativity. Oliver Sacks, neurologist and author of *Awakenings*, believes music can become a key for unlocking a sense-of-self because music can reach beyond the barriers of consciousness.

Music processing is distributed throughout several areas of the brain. This is why a specific site or sites of injury will not preclude potential benefits of music therapy. Even if language centers are damaged, you may still be able to sing! Consider that 80% of stimuli that reach our brains come in through our ears. Consider that our bodies are about 75% water. That makes them excellent conductors for sound and vibrations. Consider Deepak Chopra's explanation that atoms, cells and tissues are held together by "invisible threads" composed of vibrations.

Here are some musical suggestions from Campbell to try:

<u>Gregorian Chants</u> for relaxation, study and meditation.

<u>Slower Baroque Music</u> (Bach, Handel, Vivaldi, Corelli) for a sense of stability, order and safety. Creates a stimulating environment for study or work.

<u>Classical Music</u> (Haydn and Mozart) can improve concentration, memory and spatial perception.

<u>Jazz, Blues, Dixieland, Soul, Calypso and Reggae</u> can uplift and inspire, release joy and sadness.

<u>New Age Music</u> with no dominant rhythm elongates our sense of space and time and can induce a state of relaxed alertness.

<u>Religious and Sacred Music</u>, including shamanic drumming, church hymns, gospel music and spirituals, can ground us in the moment and lead to feelings of deep peace and spiritual awareness. It can also be remarkably useful in helping us transcend and release our pain.

Music has different effects on different people and Campbell's work is controversial. The principle behind music therapy is that different functions sometimes share the same pathways in the brain; therefore, the mastery of one activity can help enhance the performance of another.

Explore what kinds of music you enjoy and how you feel when you listen. A website or music store that has head-sets and allows you to sample music before purchasing is a good way to start if you don't have a variety at home. Check your library for rentals. Try different radio stations. I especially like Pachelbel, Tom Barabas, Rick Kuethe, George Winston and other classical or instrumental music when I'm concentrating, working at the computer, or relaxing. When I'm doing something physical like laundry or cooking and I want to feel more energetic, I like Yanni and Enya. What is most important is to discover what <u>you</u> like. *If you are hyper-sensitive to sound, try nature sounds and start at a very low volume.*

Dr. Mitchell Gaynor, author of the *Sound of Healing,* reminds us that our own voices are healing tools. Singing is a great way to tap into music's healing powers. If you like to sing, consider joining a choir. If you are self-conscious, try humming around the house. When your spirits are down, try whistling! Researchers have found that it is difficult to feel sad when you are whistling.

Movement, dance and imagery can enhance "the power of music". Dancing while seated in a chair is just as effective as dancing on your feet. Anyone can do it and **you can't do it wrong**!

Experiment and Enjoy!

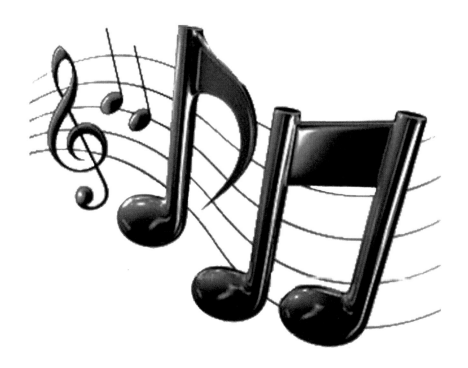

Start Small, Think Building Blocks

Strategies for Reading and Writing, Tips for Using the Computer

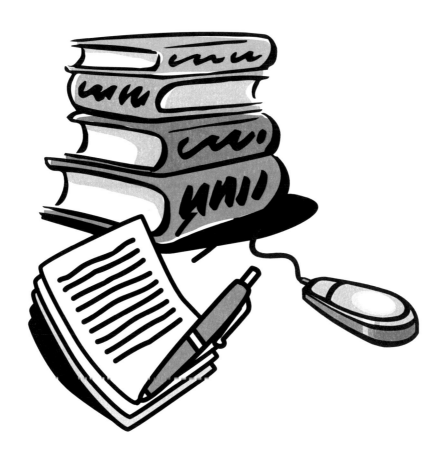

Start Small, Think Building Blocks

Strategies for Reading and Writing, Tips for Using the Computer

"The absence of words does not reflect an absence of intelligence"

— Kara Swanson
I'll Carry the Fork

Reading and writing are tasks that require a lot of focus and concentration. Plan to do these kinds of tasks at your "peak brain times" of the day and when your environment is quiet. It may be useful to go to the library for a quiet space. Set yourself up to succeed, don't even attempt it when you would likely be distracted or frequently interrupted, as is usually the case when children are home.

Work with topics that interest you as much as possible. If you are working on reading skills and you like gardening, read about gardening. If you are working on writing skills, try journaling, writing short notes to friends or thank you notes to those who have helped you since your injury.

As always, take a break when you feel fatigued, stuck or find yourself not remembering what you are reading. The more tired you feel, the longer break you need.

This chapter contains some basic strategies that may be helpful. If you continue to have problems with reading or writing, please consult a Speech and Language Pathologist. If you continue to have vision problems, please consult a visual therapist or neuro-opthamologist.

Basic Reading Strategies

<u>Start small.</u>

You can start by reading descriptions in catalogs that interest you, captions under pictures in magazines or the comics! Read one page a day in *Simple Abundance*, by Sarah Ban Breathnach. Read children's books or read to children! If it feels insulting, like you are going backwards, try to think in terms of building blocks. Sometimes you have to take a step backward in order to take two steps forward.

<u>Try using the color blue.</u>

Experiment with the lighter to medium shades to see what works best for you.

- ❏ A blue transparency to put over written material for reading
- ❏ A blue highlighter for written material
- ❏ Blue paper to write on
- ❏ A blue transparency to put over your computer screen
- ❏ Blue tinted sunglasses to work on the computer
- ❏ Blue paper to print on

<u>Use a lap desk or a pillow in your lap.</u>

Try this when you are reading so it puts material in a better position and reduces neck strain.

<u>Keep a dictionary handy to look up unfamiliar words.</u>

Don't guess or skip what you don't recognize – look it up!

<u>Consider using audio books and computer software that reads aloud to you.</u>

This can be especially helpful for lengthy material. Just remember that if you rely solely on audio books, you aren't giving yourself the opportunity to improve your reading skills.

<u>If your eyes have trouble tracking:</u>

- ❏ Try using your finger or a ruler below the line of print or a blocking guide that allows you to see one line at a time.
- ❏ Try turning your head to scan the words, instead of moving just your eyes.
- ❏ Read material in columns, like the newspaper.
- ❏ Try using large print:
    - ○ Check out the large print selections in libraries and bookstores.
    - ○ Experiment with different fonts on your computer.
    - ○ Make lists and directions in large print for easier reading.

To aid comprehension or understanding what you read:

- ❏ Read what interests you.
- ❏ Avoid novels and multiple story lines in the beginning.
- ❏ Read aloud.
- ❏ Read aloud to children!
- ❏ Try reading non-fiction books so you can read just the sections of interest. You won't have to try to follow a plot or keep track of multiple characters.
- ❏ Ask yourself if what you read makes sense. If it doesn't, think about the subject, look at any pictures, and reread it. Then ask yourself again if it makes sense.
- ❏ Stop when you feel fatigued, stuck, can't remember what you are reading or don't understand what you are reading after rereading it. Take a relaxation break or do something physical for awhile.

Recalling written material

- ❏ Use pencil marks and removable page flags to emphasize key words and help you locate important information later.
- ❏ Summarize out loud to yourself or to someone else.
- ❏ Reread to check for accuracy
- ❏ Take notes or make an outline. Use key words and doodles or sketches to create memory cues.
- ❏ Copy over your notes or outline. Repetitions always aid memory.
- ❏ When reading fiction, make a list of main characters and a brief description to help you remember who's who.

Basic Writing Strategies

<u>Stock up on pencils, erasers and a pencil sharpener!</u>

Use pencil when possible, a huge frustration saver!

<u>Try thinking and writing in key phrases.</u>

This helps you to be concise. Ask yourself, "What am I trying to say? What is my point?"

<u>Start a daily journal as soon as possible.</u>

It doesn't matter how much you write or what you write but *write in it every day.*

- ❏ Keep your journal and pencil near where you will use it, to make it convenient and help you remember.

- ❏ If you write in your journal the same time each day, the routine will help you remember to do it. I suggest every evening.

- ❏ If you are having trouble staying positive, keep a "Grateful Journal". Write at least 3 positives each day; things that made you smile that day, things that you accomplished or that went smoother than the last time you tried them. It will shift your focus and can dramatically help to shift your mood!

No matter what you write, you are working on language skills and you are creating a map of your progress that will help give you perspective when you look back on it.

<u>Keep a list of misspellings.</u>

If you tend to misspell certain words frequently, keep a list of just those words handy so you can correct them.

<u>Make an extra copy of important forms.</u>

Do this before you fill them out. Fill one out in pencil first and then copy it over in ink or photocopy the penciled version. A huge frustration saver! (Make sure you adjust the darkness of the copier to show writing in pencil.)

<u>Seeing a new doctor.</u>

Ask for any forms to be mailed to you before the appointment so you can have time to fill them out ahead of time, at home when and where you can concentrate. Having a copy of your Medical History Form (See Chapter 5.) to refer to can be a huge help here as well.

<u>Use a word processing program.</u>

Write on the computer when possible – this is another huge frustration saver!

Keep copies of all important forms and information.

It will save you a lot of anguish later if something gets lost in the system or if you're having trouble remembering what you did.

Plan time to review and proofread.

Do this the next day when you are fresh if possible or have someone else check it over for you. The bigger the project, the more lead time you will need to give yourself, to allow for "bad brain days" and time to proof read.

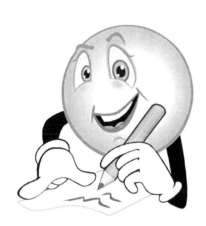

Tips for Using the Computer

Using the computer can take the torture out of writing if you are struggling. It can be a social outlet that you can access in the comfort of your home, while you are healing. You can also use it to challenge yourself with writing, doing research or playing games. However, keep in mind that if you don't practice writing by hand, your skills won't improve. Using the computer can also present new challenges as a result of your injury. You may or may not need the suggestions below, depending on your familiarity with the computer.

Safety Concerns

Keep in mind you can't believe everything you read online, on websites and in chat rooms. Consider the source.

Look for https or the padlock icon at the bottom of the page, indicating it is a secure site, before you order anything online.

Be careful about accessing any personal information like your financial data while using a public wireless access. Make sure their access is secure and can't be hijacked. Don't give out any personal information unless you know who you are "talking" to and never, never in a chat room. A good rule of thumb is don't say anything online that you wouldn't want the whole world to hear, because they just might!

Just as you may conceal your disability behind the computer, others may conceal or even misrepresent things about their identity as well. Always arrange to meet new online friends in public places. They may not turn out to be the person they presented themselves as online.

Strategies to Consider

Play with it!

You may have grown up hearing, "Don't play with it, you'll break it." You probably knew that if you broke it, you would never hear the end of it. Learning something on the computer can instantly make you feel tense and blocked. Ironically, "playing with it" is exactly how we learn these new technologies like computers and cell phones, even televisions! So try to relax, "play with it" and when you figure something out, repeat the steps a few times to help it register in your memory or write out the steps, so you can do it again!

Restore typing skills.

Try a typing tutorial to improve the speed and accuracy of your typing on the computer.

Set up a tech specialist.

A friend, relative or patient neighbor who can make a house call, in case of "techno-catastrophes".

Investigate computer classes.

They are available through libraries, adult education classes at local high schools, unemployment offices, local senior centers and disability organizations.

Repeat a class.

Expect to need to take more than one class or the same class more than once.

Learn how to use one program at a time.

The word processing program is a good place to start. It makes writing so much easier!

Write down each step.

Write it down or make a script for the most frequently used functions, including turning the computer on and off if you need to.

- ❏ You can use different colored paper or index cards for each task.
- ❏ Try large, double-spaced print for easier reading.
- ❏ Keep them together in a notebook or folder or with a ring for easy referral.

Use good computer posture.

This minimizes pain and fatigue. You may need to consult an occupational therapist or physical therapist.

Minimize eye fatigue.

- ❏ Use the computer in a well-lit room, free of glare
- ❏ Check out the accessibility and display options on your computer to make adjustments. A low contrast and a larger font are usually easier on your eyes.
- ❏ Experiment with different print styles, sizes and boldness for easy reading.
- ❏ Try using the color blue for easier reading, a light to medium shade usually works best:
    - ○ A blue transparency over your computer screen
    - ○ Blue tinted sunglasses when using the computer
    - ○ Printing on blue paper
- ❏ Look away from the computer and focus on something else every 20-30 minutes to give your eyes a break.

Remember to take breaks.

This is especially important to do when you are starting to feel pain, stuck, confused or overwhelmed. You may be able to sit at the computer for just 15 minutes at first. You can build stamina in time!

Print rough drafts to proof read.

You will read it differently on paper than you do on the computer screen.

Writing email

- ❏ Enlarge the font to apply to all emails, incoming and outgoing.
- ❏ Keep your sentences short and leave space between paragraphs.
- ❏ Fill in your address book to minimize problems from inaccurate typing and memory.

Use the favorites and bookmark features.

They help you remember frequently used websites.

All the steps needed to do something on the computer can become more automatic.

They will require less memory in time and with repetitions, like many other things we do after a brain injury.

Keep in mind that too much time on the computer is not a good thing.

You need to participate in a variety of activities to rebuild skills. The computer can contribute to feelings of isolation if you use it as a substitute for being with people.

Reward yourself for all progress, no matter how small! Don't beat yourself up for "bad brain days". You are doing the best you can at this time.

Speech and Language Pathologists are the experts to consult for help with reading and writing difficulties.

Creating a Memory Friendly System

Strategies for
Paying the Bills and Processing the Mail

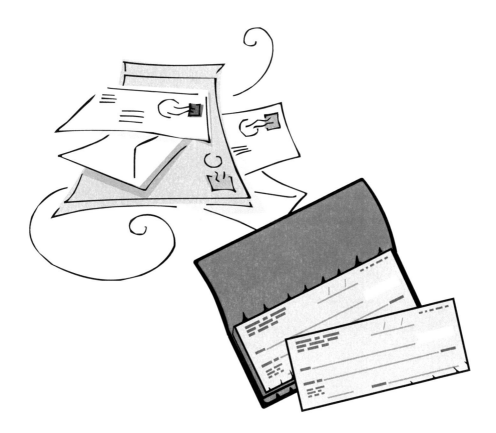

Creating A Memory Friendly System

Strategies for
Paying the Bills and Processing the Mail

"Success is to be measured not so much by the position that one has reached in life as by the obstacles which he has overcome."

— Booker T. Washington, Educator

Paying bills is one of those things you save for a "good brain day" when you can work in a "concentration friendly" environment, free of distractions and interruptions as much as possible.

General Suggestions

Sorting the mail

❏ Open the mail near the wastebasket, throwing out the obvious junk mail right away. Eliminate as much as you can, all but the "Have Tos", at least in the beginning.

❏ To deter identity theft, be sure to shred or tear up:

  ○ Any applications for loans and credit cards

  ○ Any blank checks that come with balance transfer offers

  ○ Any temporary credit cards – cut through numbers with scissors

  ○ Any personal information, including financial information, date of birth or social security numbers

❏ If you tend to go digging into the trash for things you wish you hadn't thrown out or want to check, keep a separate waste basket for mail that you empty less frequently.

❏ Cancel magazines and newspapers you don't have time to read. The more you can simplify, the easier it will be to keep up.

Master bill list

Regardless of what system you choose to pay your bills, it is a good idea to make a Master Bill List of all regular monthly bills. Keep this list with your bills. Check it against your check register at the end of the month to make sure you didn't overlook anything. (Sample at end of chapter.)

<u>Gather all the materials you will need before you begin</u>

This includes bills to pay, calculator, envelopes, stamps, pen, file for paid bills, as well as your coffee or tea so you won't get distracted or sidetracked during the process. (Refer to Chapter 7 for more suggestions on improving cognition.)

<u>Debit cards</u>

Be sure to save and record all your receipts promptly and before you pay bills. It is very easy to lose track of your bank balance. It is very costly to overdraw your bank account.

<u>Write a script</u>

If you have trouble remembering all the steps to bill paying, make a script for yourself, listing the steps. Keep it with your bills to be paid to refer to.
A possible script might be:

1. Select bill to pay according to due date

2. Write out check

3. Note check number, amount paid and date on bill receipt

4. Place payment stub and check in envelope, don't seal yet

5. Enter amount into checkbook

6. Check math with calculator

7. Repeat for each bill you need to pay

8. File receipts, now!

9. When finished, double check: make sure each check is correctly made out and you can see the mailing address on the outside of the envelope for each bill. Seal envelopes, attach stamps and return address labels.

10. Mail bills or place them where you will see them when you go out the door.

<u>If you don't trust your math:</u>

❏ Work at it.
   ○ Use your fingers if you need to
   ○ Keep your checkbook register in pencil
   ○ Check yourself with a calculator after each entry
   ○ Check your check register with the calculator again when you are finished

Working on your math can help you rebuild your math skills. If you rely solely on the calculator, you won't relearn the math.

❏ Meanwhile, have someone else check what you did before you mail the bills, until you are more sure of yourself.

❏ If you use the computer to pay bills, be sure to record all transactions in your checkbook.

<u>Leave envelopes open to double check</u>

If you find yourself wondering if you remembered to sign the check or put the right check with the right bill, leave the envelopes open so you can check them later or someone else can double check them, before mailing them.

<u>Remember to mail</u>

If you tend to forget to MAIL the bills, try putting them with your wallet and keys so you'll see them when you go out the door, or mail them as soon as you are done.

<u>Checking balances</u>

When your check register balance doesn't agree with the bank's balance, here are some things to check:

1. Check your deposit slips, ATM and debit card receipts against your register to make sure you logged them all in.

2. Did you note all automatic deposits and withdrawals?

3. Recheck your addition and subtraction with a calculator.

4. Do you have any checks outstanding? Have they all cleared or been processed by the bank?

5. Check the sequence of your check numbers to be sure you logged in all your checks. Are any numbers missing?

6. Look for any transactions that match the amount of the discrepancy. If your balance is off by $19.99, look for any entries of that amount and double check them.

7. If the difference is divisible by 9, look for numbers you might have transposed, as in 98 instead of 89.

Choosing a Weekly System or
a Daily System for Paying Bills

Weekly System

<u>Set up a "bill box" with dividers.</u>

This can be a shoebox or any similarly sized box that accommodates the standard envelope. Decorate it if you like.

1. Make dividers with any cardboard you have available. Use different colored dividers for different sections if you can. Make the dividers high enough to see a label at the top for each section.

2. Make the first section for Bills to Pay.

3. Make the following sections for paid receipts by category, Mortgage or Rent, Medical, Electric, Phone, Cable, etc.

4. You can make additional sections for Store Receipts, Pay Stubs, Bank Statements, etc. (This system keeps receipts together by category.)

<u>Paying bills</u>

1. When you receive a bill:

   ❏ Open it and check it. If you have a question about the bill, take care of it before you file it. It will make the process of paying the bills much easier.

   ❏ Mark the due date on the outside of the envelope.

   ❏ File it, in order by due date, in the first section of your Bill Box, "Bills to Pay".

2. Designate a day each week to pay bills for the week. Mark your planner/calendar to remind you of "bill day". Make it the same day each week when possible, to help you remember to do it.

3. At the end of the month, check your Master Bill List against your check register entries to make sure you haven't missed anything.

Daily System

Purchase an expandable file, with sections numbered 1-31 for days of the month and an additional section for each month.

<u>Paying bills</u>

1. When you receive a bill:
   - ❏ Open it, check it and mark the due date on the outside of the envelope.
   - ❏ Put the bill in the 1-31 file under the date you need to <u>send</u> it out, usually <u>7 days before the due date</u>.
   - ❏ If the bill is due the next month, put it in the section for that month.

2. Check your file every day, make it part of your daily routine. On the first of the month, check section #1 (for the first day of the month). On the second day of the month, check section #2 (for the second day of the month).
   - ❏ If there is a bill to pay, write out your check. On the portion of the bill that you will file, make a note of the check number, amount and date paid.
   - ❏ Place the paid receipt behind the current month in the expandable file. (Receipts will be organized by month paid.)
   - ❏ Repeat every day, (always working about 7 days before the actual date).

3. Near the end of the month, day 25 or 26, transfer all of the bills in the section for the next month, on to the next month by appropriate dates, <u>7 days before the due date</u>.

4. Check your Master Bill List against your checkbook entries at the end of the month to make sure you haven't missed anything.

NOTE: *This daily system can also be used for any time sensitive materials.*
If you get a reminder for a meeting you'd like to attend, mark the date in your Planner/Calendar and then put the information behind that date in the file. If you will need to get materials ready for a meeting, pre-register or arrange transportation, file it 3-4 days ahead of the due date.

Establishing a system for paying bills and making it part of your routine will help you remember to do it. You can also leave yourself reminders on your calendars or in your planners.

Maintaining detailed records and balancing your check register every month is the only way to know exactly what is in your account. Remember, the bank's balance on a given day does not account for outstanding checks or any automatic transactions. Accurate record keeping will alert you to any discrepancies on your behalf or the bank's. It is often wise to consider overdraft protection as a safety net. Overdraft fees can mount up very quickly.

If bill paying feels too difficult, frustrating or overwhelming, consider delegating it to someone else, at least temporarily. Healing is a process. You may be able to do this at a later time, even if it feels impossible now

Paying bills is not an easy task! Remember to take a break and reward yourself in some way when you are finished!

Master Bill List

1. List all regular monthly bills in order by due date.
2. Check it off after it is paid.
3. Compare to check register at end of month.

Bills	Jan	Feb	Mar	Apr	May	June	July	Aug	Sept	Oct	Nov	Dec

Notes

Simplify, Get Organized, Start Early

Strategies for Meal Planning, Shopping and Cooking

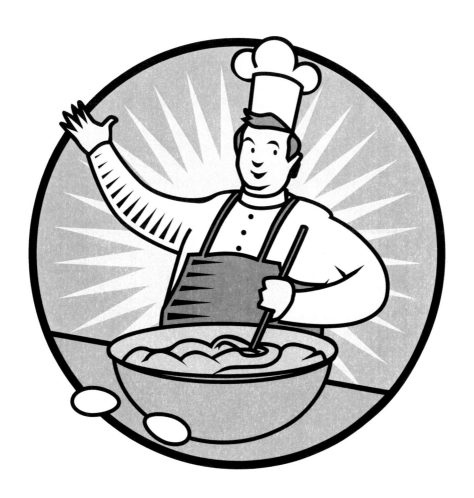

Simplify, Get Organized, Start Early

Strategies for Meal Planning, Shopping and Cooking

"There is no progress without failure. And each failure is a lesson learned."

— David Bowie, Musician

Meal Planning: Simplify as Much as Possible.

Let it be OK to simplify.

It's OK not to serve the elaborate meals you used to and use paper plates and cups. Try not to let simplifying feel like failure. Think of it as a rehabilitation strategy. Remember, you are healing and your energy is limited. Doesn't it make more sense to have a simple, peaceful meal than to fall apart trying to prepare a complicated one?

Stock up on prepared foods for standbys.

This is really helpful for those days when you are too tired to cook or having a "bad brain" day.

- ❏ Keep some frozen dinners, vegetables and entrées on hand. There is a wide variety available in the freezer section of the grocery store these days.
- ❏ Keep staples on hand that have a long shelf life: canned vegetables and fruits, soups, cereals, pastas, rice, tuna, cheese, eggs and peanut butter.
- ❏ Keep breads in the freezer for extended shelf life.

Use a crockpot and make "one pot" meals.

Soups, stews and casseroles are easy.

Pick up a pre-prepared main dish.

You can find this at the grocery store. Add salad and bread or a couple of veggies and you have a meal! You can even use the grocery store's salad bar or packaged salad mixes.

Sandwiches can be fun!

Purchase a variety of breads and rolls, fillings and garnishes and let family members make their own. Add fruit, salad or a cup of soup and you have a full meal.

Plan an easy meal for busy days and your shopping day.

You can do this any day you expect to be especially tiring. This is where you can use those items you stocked up. Let it be a "microwave magic night" or make it "whatever you want night" and everyone is on their own! It could also be "take out night".

Conquering Grocery Shopping!

Begin by writing down a few ideas for meals.

- ❏ Check your pantry and freezer for possibilities.
- ❏ Check the grocery store flyer for sale items and ideas.
- ❏ Check your recipes for ingredients needed.
- ❏ Add needed items to your shopping list.

Master grocery shopping list (Sample at end of chapter)

Suggestions for modifying to suit your needs:

- ❏ Rearrange categories to match the order of your favorite store.
- ❏ Write in your staples; the items you usually shop for each week.
- ❏ Make copies for additional weeks.
- ❏ Post in the kitchen, add items as you get low or run out. Instruct your family to do so as well!

If weekly grocery shopping is overwhelming …

- ❏ You may need to plan one day and shop the next day or
- ❏ You may need to plan meals and shop for just 2 days at a time.

Gather everything you will need to go grocery shopping.

Place items near your purse/wallet where you will see them when you go out the door.

- ❏ Grocery shopping list, coupons (optional) and store flyer. They will help your memory.
- ❏ Method of payment
- ❏ Sunglasses or cap and earplugs if they are helpful.
- ❏ Yellow tinted glasses if helpful with fluorescent lights.
- ❏ Bottles and cans to return, bags to recycle, reusable shopping bags

Have a snack.

Do this before you leave if you haven't eaten in awhile to keep your energy up and impulse buying down.

Shop when the stores are the quietest.

This is usually early in the week and early in the day, before 2:00 p.m. if possible. Avoid weekends.

Shop just one store.

It will be less confusing, less fatiguing and you will get to know the store better.

Park your car in the same general area of the parking lot.

If possible, park in the same area each time you go to that store. It will help you locate your car later.

Use a carriage.

Even if you only need a few things, using a carriage is less taxing than carrying things and it gives you something to lean on for balance.

Use a clipboard.

Check off items as you put them in your cart.

Ask for help.

If you are having trouble locating items, ask at the Customer Service Dept. for a store map or a list of items by aisle. Sometimes these lists are hanging on the end of the aisles. If a store map or list of items by aisle is not available, create your own! (Sample at end of chapter which you can modify to match your store as closely as possible.)

Keep frozen and refrigerator items together.

This makes it easier to unload just those items and put them away if you are too tired to do it all when you get home.

Ask for help unloading the groceries.

Children? Neighbor children?

Delegate the job of putting the groceries away.

Ask others in your household to help.

Delegate shopping.

Ask a family member if it is practical.

Plan "down time" after shopping and an easy supper.

I make sure I pick up a frozen pizza and salad on grocery shopping day!

Consider using a food service or a "milk man".

Some large grocers offer this service; ask about any extra charge.
It may be worth it for you.

Cooking: Start Early, Take it One Step at a Time

Early in the day

Do this early in the day before noon. Figure out what you want to eat for supper, especially if you have a family to cook for.

❑ Try to anticipate your energy level: are you going to be busy and probably need something simple for supper or do you anticipate an easier day with time and energy to cook?

❑ Check your recipe. Can you locate it? Do you need to write it out?

❑ Check ingredients on the recipe. Do you have what you need? Will you need to pick something up from the store?

❑ Figure out when you will need to *start* preparations in order to give yourself enough time to work at your own pace and in an organized manner.

Take a recharging rest break **before** you start dinner.

This is probably **the** most important strategy for a successful meal. It takes energy and concentration to cook and you've already had a full day. People without health problems have difficulties managing this time of day, especially with children. Pushing too hard can result in a disaster, instead of a dinner!

Minimize distractions and interruptions.

Let the machine answer the phone. Get the kids quieted down doing homework or watching TV. Have children use headphones for their music and the TV if you are having trouble screening out the sounds.

Plan extra time.

Figure on at least **double** the time you used to, work at your own pace and *do one thing at a time.* For example:

❑ Begin by setting the table.

❑ Next make the salad, wash and cut up vegetables or fruit.

❑ Then start cooking whatever will need to cook the longest.

  ○ Avoid cooking more than one thing at a time on the stove.

  ○ Use the microwave when possible.

  Exception: if you are using a crockpot or making a slow-cooking meal like a stew, you will need to start cooking that first, early in the day.

❑ Delegate the table setting and making the salad, if it won't cause too much confusion for you.

❑ Delegate cleanup if it is practical.

Timing meals

If you have trouble timing meals so everything is ready at the same time, please refer to Reverse Scheduling in Chapter 6. You can use the same method as you do for figuring out how to get to appointments on time. This time the "appointment" is your meal.

Other time and energy saving tips

❏ Cook double the amount and freeze half of it. You will have a treat to pull out of the freezer on one of those days when you are too tired to cook. (Remember to label and date containers.)

❏ Cook enough pasta or rice for 2 days. Serve it hot with meat sauce for one meal. Make a pasta salad the next day with leftover vegetables and meats mixed in for a second meal.

❏ Make the salad or main dish earlier in the day, maybe before the kids get home, to simplify the process later.

❏ Sit to chop or peel fruits and vegetables, when possible, to conserve energy.

❏ Leave the skin on vegetables like carrots and potatoes for less work and more vitamins when it is practical, like when you make something like a stew. Be sure to wash them thoroughly.

❏ Try cooking bags or line pans with a double layer of aluminum foil to make clean up easier.

❏ Use paper plates and paper cups.

❏ Consider serving food directly from pots rather than moving it to serving dishes and creating more dishes to wash.

❏ Air-dry dishes instead of hand drying.

❏ For social occasions when you need to take a food item, remember you don't have to *make* it; you just need to *take* it. There is a large variety of prepared food available for take-out and in the grocery stores these days.

Trouble finding or remembering your favorite recipes?

Suggestions:

❏ Make frequently used recipes easier to find by checking or underlining them in the index of the cookbook. Use removable page flags or Post It® notes on the recipe page.

❏ Make notes (in pencil) in the margins for any changes that you usually make when using a recipe.

❏ Make a notebook of favorite recipes. This becomes your personal cookbook!

<u>Trouble following recipes?</u>

Suggestions:

- ❏ Check out the different kinds of cookbooks that are available:
    - ○ Picture cookbooks
    - ○ Five ingredient cookbooks
    - ○ Slow-cooker cookbooks
- ❏ Write out favorite recipes in **LARGE PRINT.**
- ❏ Before you start, pull out all the ingredients and utensils you will need for the recipe. As you add each ingredient, put it away.
- ❏ Use a pencil to check off each ingredient as you add it and each step as you complete it.
- ❏ Use an extra large (12 cup) measuring cup so you can tell how many cups you have measured out for a recipe.

<u>Trouble remembering something is in the oven?</u>

- ❏ Stay in the kitchen and work on something else or take a rest break while using the oven so your nose will help you remember.
- ❏ Carry the timer with you if you leave the room or
- ❏ Use the kind of timer that you can wear around your neck.
- ❏ **Make sure you have working smoke detectors!**

<u>If you have trouble remembering to shut things off:</u>

- ❏ Post a list to check when you finish cooking.
- ❏ Make that checklist part of your routine when you leave the house or go to bed.
- ❏ Have another family member double check to make sure everything is shut off after the meal or before going to bed.
- ❏ Use the microwave instead of the stove as much as possible.
- ❏ **Make sure you have working smoke detectors!**

Helpful tips

Sometimes the best strategy is to SIMPLIFY as much as possible, at least initially.

Let it be OK to ask for and accept help. Delegate what you can. This may be very hard for you if you are used to "doing it all".

If delegating feels too confusing, try making a list ahead of time of the things you could use help with. Then you can make assignments from the list or you can ask volunteers to choose the tasks they would like to help with.

For more help with meal planning, shopping and cooking, consult an occupational therapist.

Meal Ideas

Monday

Breakfast

Lunch

Dinner

Tuesday

Breakfast

Lunch

Dinner

Wednesday

Breakfast

Lunch

Dinner

Thursday

Breakfast

Lunch

Dinner

Friday

Breakfast

Lunch

Dinner

Saturday

Breakfast

Lunch

Dinner

Sunday

Breakfast

Lunch

Dinner

Tools

Master Grocery Shopping List

Fresh Fruits and Vegetables

- ❏ _____
- ❏ _____
- ❏ _____
- ❏ _____

Meats, Fish, Deli

- ❏ _____
- ❏ _____
- ❏ _____
- ❏ _____

Staples Soup, pasta, rice, canned goods

- ❏ _____
- ❏ _____
- ❏ _____
- ❏ _____

Cereals Oatmeal, bran mix

- ❏ _____
- ❏ _____
- ❏ _____
- ❏ _____

Baking Sugar, flour, cake mix

- ❏ _____
- ❏ _____
- ❏ _____
- ❏ _____

Beverages Coffee, tea, soda

- ❏ _____
- ❏ _____
- ❏ _____
- ❏ _____

Snacks Popcorn, crackers, cookies, Jello

- ❏ _____
- ❏ _____
- ❏ _____
- ❏ _____

Paper Plates, napkins, towels, toilet paper

- ❏ _____
- ❏ _____
- ❏ _____
- ❏ _____

Dairy Milk, eggs, cheese, yogurt, juice

- ❏ _____
- ❏ _____
- ❏ _____
- ❏ _____

Frozen Pizza, vegetables

- ❏ _____
- ❏ _____
- ❏ _____
- ❏ _____

Breads, Baked Goods

- ❏ _____
- ❏ _____
- ❏ _____
- ❏ _____

Cleaning Dish soap, laundry detergent

- ❏ _____
- ❏ _____
- ❏ _____
- ❏ _____

Personal Soap, shampoo, toothpaste

- ❏ _____
- ❏ _____
- ❏ _____
- ❏ _____

Other Pet food, batteries, light bulbs, etc

- ❏ _____
- ❏ _____
- ❏ _____
- ❏ _____

Tools

Sample Grocery Store Map

Write in the items you need to shop for

Meats, Fish, Deli

Ground Beef
Bacon
Chicken

Fresh Fruits and Vegetables

Lettuce
Tomato
Apples
Bananas

Pantry Staples

Soup
Pasta
Rice
Cereal

Baking Supplies

Sugar
Flour

Beverages Snacks

Sodas
Popcorn
Chips

Paper Goods Cleaning Supplies

Tissue
Towels
Detergent
Trash bags

Frozen Foods

Pizza
Ice Cream

Dairy

Milk
Yogurt
Eggs
Cheese
Juice

Cashiers

Door

Door

Tools

Tools

Grocery Store Map

Write in the aisle headings that pertain to your store and then the items you need to shop for

Door

Cashiers

Door

Saving Your Energy

Strategies for Shopping, Errands and Gift Giving

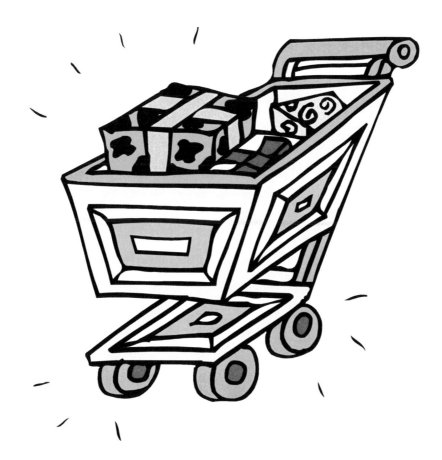

Saving Your Energy

Strategies for Shopping, Errands and Gift Giving

"The only people who always remember where they parked their cars are people who always park in the same area of the parking lot"

— Gary Small
The Memory Bible

Shopping and doing errands are an enormous energy drain. This is the time to delegate, to take family and friends up on their offers of help. Think of it as giving them an opportunity to feel helpful. Conserve your energy for your healing as much as possible.

Helpful Suggestions

Consider your overall energy and pacing needs for the week.

Plan to shop when you can take it easy the next day, or two, to recuperate. Stock up on prepared foods for standbys.

Plan to shop when the stores will be less congested.

This is usually early in the week and early in the day. Friday nights can be OK but avoid weekends.

Take your list, earplugs, cap or sunglasses, store card and method of payment.

Park your car in the same general area.

Use the same area of the parking lot each time you go to a particular store. This will help you remember where it is. You can also leave yourself a message on your cell phone or make a note on your shopping list.

Use a carriage when possible.

Even if you only need a few things, using a carriage is less tiring than carrying a basket or individual items. It also gives you something to lean on and can be helpful with balance.

Plan to take breaks.

You'll be surprised how much it helps to take a few minutes for water, coffee or tea, a snack or just to sit and rest. Think of taking a break as a "performance strategy". If taking a break doesn't help, it is time to go home!

Organize your shopping list by store or by categories.

❏ <u>By store</u> if you plan to shop just one store for multiple items. Make a list of everything you want to look for while you are in that store.

❏ <u>By category</u> if you plan to shop more than one store and you are not sure where you will find the items. Make your list by categories of items you need to look for: clothing, health and beauty items, stationery supplies, household items, etc.

Clothes shopping

Make a detailed list. Check your closets first and make a note of what you have and what you are looking for, including sizes and colors. This is especially important if you shop for more than one person. You may find it helpful to keep a list of sizes for basic items in your purse or planner.

Grocery shopping

See Chapter 10 on Meal Planning, Shopping and Cooking.

If you find yourself overwhelmed, break your shopping down into manageable chunks.

Shop for one or two items at a time, like when you need to comparison shop for clothes.

Shop one or two stores at a time, when you need numerous items.

Plan your shopping to avoid backtracking and save energy.

Prioritize and plan your route to avoid extra driving.
Consult a map if it will be helpful.

❏ Are there any "Must Do's" on your list? Start there.

❏ If there are no "Must Do's" on your list, start with the store farthest away from home. Then if you get overtired and aren't able to complete your list, you will be closer to home.

Use mall maps if you are going to a mall, to help you figure out how to save yourself steps. Malls are designed to keep you there, not to save steps!

Consider shopping from catalogs and online.

This helps when you trust the quality of the store or website and know your sizes in specific brands. It can be a huge time and energy saver. However:

❏ Returning unwanted items can create another job for you and an additional expense.

❏ Be sure to use only secure sites indicated with a padlock symbol beside the address bar.

❏ Pay particular attention to details like delivery. You don't want an expensive item left on your doorstep when you are not home, to be potentially stolen.

Gift Giving - Keeping it Simple

Gift giving was a big problem for me. I didn't have the money to spend on gifts or the energy to do everything I used to do. I agonized and struggled to keep up until I began to dread special occasions. Finally I decided it was time to figure out how to bring some joy back into the holidays. If you are struggling in this area, I hope you will find some of the following suggestions helpful.

Cut back.

Where you can, at least temporarily. Explain to friends and relatives ahead of time. Let it be OK to cut back. Isn't it better to do less and be able to enjoy it, than to try to do more or spend more than is reasonable for you at this time and not be able to enjoy it? Would your family or friends want to receive a gift that you didn't enjoy giving?

Start early.

Give yourself a lot of lead-time, especially if you need to mail something.

Consider substituting.

Think of something else that is less taxing and more meaningful for you, perhaps a birthday phone call, or a get together for coffee.

Use one general idea for several people.

Examples might be baking cookies for your friends or knitting scarves for family.

Use gift certificates or bank gift cards.

You can create your own gift certificates for something you would like to spend time doing together, maybe a movie or playing scrabble.

Purchase greeting cards monthly.

Before the beginning of the month, for birthdays and other special occasions. **Consider sending free email cards.**

Holiday cards:

- ❏ Make your own cards using the computer, your own artwork or a favorite photo.
- ❏ Let it be OK to send just a few cards, maybe there are people who were especially helpful the past year.
- ❏ Consider sending cards for Thanksgiving or Valentine's Day, instead of in December.
- ❏ Let it be OK not to send any cards when you wouldn't enjoy doing it. Many healthy people don't send out holiday cards.

<u>Use catalogs or shop online.</u>

This helps to get ideas or to have items sent directly to recipients to eliminate shopping, wrapping and mailing! Shop catalogs and websites you are familiar with, trust and can depend on their quality.

<u>Have items gift wrapped while you are shopping.</u>

Look for charities that have tables set up and will do it inexpensively.

<u>Gift bags and tissue paper are easier than wrapping paper.</u>

Look for inexpensive supplies in craft stores and discount stores.

<u>Let it be ok, give yourself permission, to let go of traditions that don't work now.</u>

Maybe it is a good time to start a new, easier and meaningful tradition. Have a family meeting before the holidays and decide together what is most important, what you can let go of and what you can simplify. Hold on to the traditions that mean the most to you.

I loved to bake lots of cookies, from scratch, for the holidays. After my injury, when my son was small, I knew I had to find an easier way or give it up all together. So I purchased cookie dough that I could slice, we pressed them with the bottom of a decorative glass to make a fancy pattern and sprinkled them with sugar. My son was thrilled and I didn't feel like I had to give up yet another thing that was important to me.

"The excellence of a gift lies in its appropriateness rather than its value."

— Charles Dudley Warner, Writer

Memory Jogger List and Plan for Errands

(Remember to check your calendar or planner as well.)

Errands

- ❏ Bank
- ❏ Post Office
- ❏ Gas
- ❏ Grocery Store
- ❏ Pharmacy
- ❏ Greeting Card/Gift Store
- ❏ Library
- ❏ Dry Cleaners
- ❏ Video Store
- ❏ _____
- ❏ _____
- ❏ _____
- ❏ _____
- ❏ _____
- ❏ _____
- ❏ _____
- ❏ _____
- ❏ _____
- ❏ _____
- ❏ _____
- ❏ _____

My Plan

Monday
_____
_____
_____

Tuesday
_____
_____
_____

Wednesday
_____
_____
_____

Thursday
_____
_____
_____

Friday
_____
_____
_____

Saturday
_____
_____
_____

Sunday
_____
_____
_____

Arrange your list by:

Priority, when there are "Must Dos" – start there

Travel distance, when there are no "Must Dos".

Remember to take a break in a quiet place when you <u>start</u> to feel fatigued. If it doesn't recharge you, it is time to go home or take a nap in your car.

Tools

Creating Space

Strategies for Conquering Clutter

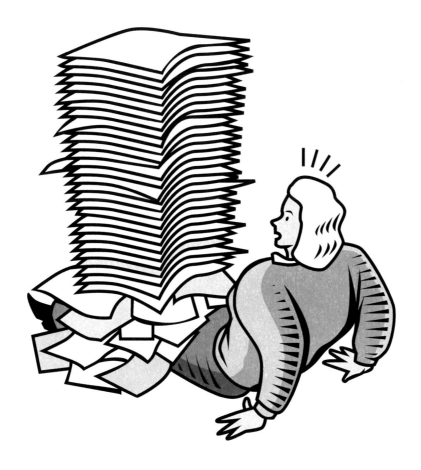

Creating Space

Strategies for Conquering Clutter

Here are four old-fashioned rules for bringing order into your home. Post them in every room. Teach them to your children. Whisper them in your partner's ear.

> *If you take it out, put it back.*
>
> *If you open it, close it.*
>
> *If you throw it down, pick it up.*
>
> *If you take it off, hang it up.*

— Sarah Ban Breathnach
Simple Abundance

Clutter is a huge problem for almost everyone who has health problems. While you are out of commission from an illness or injury, the clutter accumulates. This issue is compounded for people with brain injury because you are working with compromised cognitive processing skills that make it harder to handle anything at all! On top of that, survivors of brain injury also have two kinds of clutter to deal with, physical clutter and clutter of the mind. No wonder we feel confused, overwhelmed, stressed and out of control! It is mind-boggling. It feels impossible!

I think the best advice I can give you is to <u>prevent</u> as much clutter as possible. Face the fact that you can't do as much as you used to right now. You <u>have to</u> simplify your life as much as possible. Focus on allowing only what is absolutely necessary into your life. This applies to physical items like the mail, things you have to do and things you need to think about. It is survival, or "healing mode", for now.

Working in an organized, clutter free space helps you focus and think better, especially if you have visual processing problems. There is less to distract you. Staying organized helps your memory. You know where to find things. This chapter contains some suggestions that I hope will help you to conquer your clutter and keep it that way!

TIP #1 Prevent as Much Clutter as You Can.

<u>Stop any unnecessary newspapers and magazines.</u>

Get rid of those that aren't read, piling up and are making you feel frustrated.

<u>Throw out as much mail as you can, as you sort it.</u>

This includes all junk mail, solicitations, catalogs you won't use, etc.

- ❏ Keep only what is absolutely necessary. Ask yourself: "Do I have to tend to this?" You'll be surprised at how much you can eliminate!

- ❏ Remember to destroy personal information and any blank credit applications, blank checks or temporary credit cards.

- ❏ If you find yourself digging through the trash for things you're afraid you threw away in error, keep a separate trash basket for sorting the mail and doing paperwork. Empty it less often.

<u>Whenever updated material arrives, throw out the old version.</u>

For example:

- ❏ When you file a new insurance policy, throw out the old one.

- ❏ When a new phone book is delivered, recycle the old one.

- ❏ When a new catalog arrives, recycle the old one.

  (See "Recommended Documents to Keep" at the end of this chapter)

<u>You will probably need to stop most extracurricular activities and hobbies for now.</u>

This applies to anything that will create another job for you. For example, you may want to suspend taking photographs if you know it will be difficult to follow through labeling and organizing them, thus creating another source of frustration and clutter! You may want to do your gardening in containers for the time being, instead of trying to manage a regular garden plot.

<u>Simplify your life as much as possible, for now.</u>

This is a good time to reevaluate your family/birthday/holiday commitments. Talk to your family about your concerns and intentions.

This was very hard for me. I didn't want to let others down. I felt like I had failed, but I couldn't keep up with everything. Special occasions were making me angry and broke, instead of bringing me joy. Finally taking this step to cut back and simplify was very liberating for me. My family was happy that I was happier.

<u>Be very careful what you agree to or volunteer for.</u>

It is OK to say, "I'm sorry, I can't right now." No further explanation is necessary, especially to telephone solicitors!

<u>Try not to take on any new projects or commitments.</u>

Wait until you feel like you are managing what you have to.

TIP #2 Try to Handle Things Only Once.

<u>When you sort the mail.</u>

Eliminate as much as you can, then label and put the bills away in your bill file *right away*.

<u>When you unpack bags, put the items away.</u>

Put them where they belong, right away. However there are exceptions:

❏ If you are too tired after shopping, put away any perishable items and then take a break. Delegate if you can.

❏ If you need to put things away on another floor, you can save energy by collecting items for that floor near the stairs. Then put all of those items away at the same time the next time you go upstairs. Delegate if you can.

❏ Resist, as hard as you can, just putting things down anywhere or you will soon have clutter everywhere. If you are too tired and need to take a break, try your best to get back to it before the end of the day.

TIP #3 Create Zones.

Examples:

❏ A Drop Zone ... near the door for keys, wallet and cell phone, outdoor clothes, backpacks. Use baskets, boxes, shelves, hooks.

❏ Collection Zones ... for sports equipment, music, videos, etc.

❏ Schoolwork Zones ... folders or small boxes of different colors to collect each child's papers.

❏ A Bill Zone... an area where you keep your bills, file for paid receipts, calculator, pens, stamps ... everything you'll need when you pay the bills. You'll be less likely to create piles to file later if you have everything you need close at hand.

<u>Use any organization systems that you already have in place.</u>

Build on existing systems with labels and containers rather than creating a new system. It is easier to follow a system that has already been established than it is to remember a completely new system.

TIP #4 Help getting started

❏ Begin by planning the reward - for when you are finished!

❏ What area bothers you the most? That is where you start.

❏ Try putting on some peppy music softly in the background.

❏ Try starting with a bag for trash and going around the house collecting all the trash first, then the dirty dishes, dirty laundry, etc.

❏ Feeling overwhelmed or stuck? Break your project down into smaller parts. Take it one step at a time.

❏ Make a list of "mini-jobs" that take 10 minutes or less. Small jobs, done well, can be a huge motivator!

❏ Ask a friend to help. Committing to a day and a time to start and having someone else for moral support can be a really big help!

<u>Make a plan to catch up on accumulated clutter.</u>

Set aside all the time you have for one week; or one day each week, like every Saturday, until you catch up.

Hang in there, things didn't get messy in one day. Once you have caught up and created a place or zone for everything you will find it cleans up much faster, even when you haven't been able to keep up with it consistently.

TIP #5 Deciding What to Keep and What to Let Go of. Ask Yourself:

"Is it a pain in the heart or a pain in the butt?
If it is a pain in the heart – keep it or do something about it.
If it is a pain in the butt – why hold on to it?"

— Craig, survivor

(Refer to "Recommended Documents to Keep" at the end of this chapter)

TIP #6 Maintenance

<u>There are two basic keys for managing clutter:</u>

❏ Prevent as much as possible.

❏ Tend to it regularly; schedule it into your daily and weekly routine.

If you can follow these two concepts, managing your clutter will be the most difficult only in the beginning, when you are digging out and getting reorganized. It is a lot easier to keep up than it is to catch up.

<u>Establish routine times for tending to accumulated clutter.</u>

Every day at 4:00, before supper, might be a good time. Maybe Saturday mornings are better for you.

<u>If you have children, be sure they help!</u>

Give specific 15-minute directions like, "Please gather up all the dirty clothes" and then, "Please gather up the dirty dishes." Tie it into a fun thing, "When we get the work done we can …"

<u>If you find that the clutter keeps accumulating:</u>

You need to do one of two things. Spend more time on maintenance or simplify your life more.

See "Blueprint for Conquering Clutter" at the end of this chapter for a strategy to help you dig out of accumulated clutter. Think about someone to give you a hand with this. Most survivors I know who are successful at managing their clutter have had help - a friend, family member or a professional organizer.

Reward all accomplishments!

Blueprint for Conquering Clutter
(Start small - a pile, a corner, a drawer.)

#1 SEPARATE items into three piles:

Saves   Discards   Unsure

#2 SORT through Unsure pile, move to:

Saves	or	Discards
❏ Use currently		❏ Out of date
❏ Has meaning		❏ Not used in last year
❏ Permanent document		❏ No room for
		(Can you take a photo instead?)

#3 ORGANIZE Saves

Put "like items" together.

#4 CONTAINERIZE and DESIGNATE

Storage areas for SAVES, putting "like items" together. Be as creative as you like! Use cardboard boxes, clear plastic containers, boxes covered with contact paper, baskets with ribbons, colored folders. Be sure to label containers, shelves and drawers.

#5 ELIMINATE Discards

Donate, Yard Sale, Recycle, Trash

Congratulations! Do a victory dance!
Reward yourself! Plan your next area to conquer!

Recommended Documents to Keep

❏ Tax Records – 3 yrs for personal and self employment, 7 yrs for business

❏ Bank Statements, Cancelled Checks – 7 yrs

❏ Marriage, Birth and Death Certificates

❏ Settlement and Divorce Papers

❏ Adoption, Custody, Citizenship and Military Papers

❏ Trust Papers, Living Will, Power of Attorney

❏ Property Deeds, Motor Vehicle Titles

❏ Stock and Bond Certificates

❏ U.S. Savings Bonds

❏ All Contracts and any Legal Documents

❏ Home Inventory List, Photos, Receipts for Valuables, Appraisals

❏ Receipts for "Big Ticket" Items

❏ Yearly Calendars/Planners – for memory joggers and disability reviews

NOTE: Store important financial and legal documents in a safe-deposit box or a fire-safe box.

Starting Over

Strategies for Social Situations

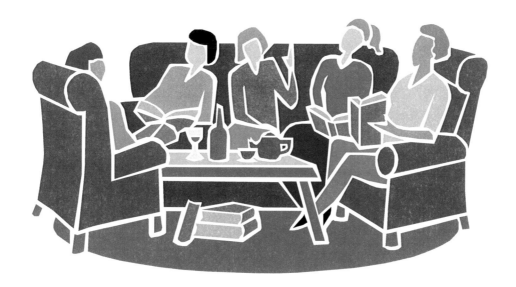

Starting Over

Strategies for Social Situations

"Imagine that every person in the world is enlightened but you. They are all your teachers, each doing just the right things to help you learn patience, perfect wisdom, perfect compassion."

— Buddha

Building social connections is as important as rebuilding cognitive skills after a brain injury. A social network promotes a sense of belonging and confidence, which supports learning.

However, this is no easy task. Many of your former friends may not be available, especially if your social network was mainly work-related and you are no longer working. You cannot enjoy the same activities you used to. People can be impatient and cruel. Awareness is increasing about brain injury but the general public's knowledge is still limited. You may be struggling with changes, deficits and low tolerances as a result of your injury. You may not know what to say to people about what happened to you. You may feel wounded and fragile. You may feel "ambushed" when you run into something you didn't anticipate. Panic can set in.

No wonder we tend to isolate after a brain injury! It is a very scary and painful place to be. I think planning for and anticipating situations is key but it takes time to know what to expect and to figure out how to accommodate your new set of needs. It is trial and error at first, a discovery process. Try to be patient with yourself and others. The following sections offer some suggestions that I hope you will find helpful.

Safety First: Staying Out of Trouble

A common problem after a brain injury is impaired judgment, which makes it difficult to figure out what is safe and sensible, especially in social situations. Your decision-making difficulties may be compounded by lack of awareness and impulsivity as a result of your brain injury. You may also be feeling isolated since your injury and longing for social interaction. Those feelings alone may give you the tendency to make poor decisions.

Your first hint that your judgment may be impaired may be a sinking feeling in your gut. Or it may be when you encounter resistance from family members when you want to do something that they don't think is wise. Try to listen to that feeling in your gut and trust that your family has your best interest in mind when they raise concerns. If you have the awareness that your judgment may not be intact, try to accept it for now and make a habit of talking things over with a friend, family member or therapist, before you do something new since your injury.

If you are a parent, maintain good communication with your co-parent about what is going on with your children. If a co-parent isn't available, run the issue in question by a friend or another parent before you say yes to your child. It can be difficult to resist but don't let your child pressure you into a quick decision that you aren't comfortable with. Just say you need time to think about it; you want to make a good decision for both of you. It will never be wrong to wait, it may be very wrong to give permission in haste. It may make sense to work with a family therapist or social worker for awhile.

Some of the typically risky situations to be aware of and seek guidance about are:

Driving

This is an extremely dangerous and complex task. You may still have your license but it doesn't mean you should be driving, yet. See Chapter 14 for more discussion on this topic.

Alcohol and substance abuse

This is risky behavior that impairs your judgment. This was true before your injury and it is a very, very, very bad idea after an injury. It will complicate and slow your rehabilitation. Keep in mind your brain chemistry has changed since your injury and 1 alcoholic drink = 3 alcoholic drinks! The last thing you need after a brain injury is something that will impair your cognition and judgment even more.

Internet dating and chat rooms

On the Internet, anyone can be anyone they want to be. Never give out any personal information like your social security or credit card numbers, your address or phone number.

Meeting someone new

Always meet someone new in a public place where there will be other people around if you find you feel uncomfortable. Never let a stranger pick you up or take you home. Take a friend with you if you can, for safety and moral support.

Places where others are engaging in risky behaviors

This includes parties, bar rooms and concerts. It can be easy to get swept up or involved in risky behaviors, even if you didn't intend to. Stay away until you have experienced enough social situations successfully that you feel confident you will be comfortable and safe.

Friends

True friends will have your best interest at heart. They may not understand all your issues but they will not want you to do something that makes you uncomfortable. Unfortunately, not all friends are true friends. You may lose some "friends". You may gain some truer friends.

As you heal, you will naturally want to return to as much of your normal life as possible. If you have had difficulties with your judgment, you may need to rebuild it, like other skills. Some of the worksheets at the end of this chapter may be helpful.

Attend social situations with family and friends in the beginning, while you are figuring out how to be comfortable in different situations so they can assist you if needed.

There may be times, many times, when **not** participating in an activity is good judgment and is your best decision. If you know that crowds and loud sounds are hard for you to tolerate for example, it may be best for you to skip the shopping trip to the mall. If you are wondering if an activity is a "risky behavior", make a habit of asking yourself three things:

1. What is the worst thing that could happen?
2. What could I do about it if the worst thing did happen?
3. What would the end result be?

When you have had successful social events, you will gain confidence and your family will gain confidence in you. If you find that you continue to have difficulties in this area, it may be helpful to work with a social worker or behavioral therapist.

General Suggestions for Social Situations:

<u>Think about disclosure.</u>

Most survivors struggle with this issue a lot. What will you say to people who haven't seen you in awhile when they ask, "What happened?" "Where have you been?" or "How are you?" Reactions will vary and may surprise you. Keeping your answer brief usually works best until you can gauge their level of genuine interest.

Giving up on the expectation that other people could understand what I was going through is what helped me with this issue. Most people aren't able to understand it, not because they don't want to and not because they aren't good people. They just don't have the necessary life experience to understand it. It is similar to not being able to understand what it is like to live with cancer or another serious illness if you haven't had that experience.

Once I gave up expecting people to understand, I could give up on the struggle of trying to make them understand and eliminate the frustration when they didn't "get it". I explain things as simply as I can and let it go. Some key phrases I like to use are, "I was in a car accident a while ago and I had to take some time off to heal" or "I've been dealing with some health issues" or "I have to write everything down since my car accident (surgery/stroke), would you mind repeating that, please?"

<u>Surround yourself with supportive people as much as possible.</u>

If there are difficult people in your family or community, minimize your involvement with them as much as possible for now. Remember, you are healing and you need your energy for healing.

<u>Spiritual supports in your life are important.</u>

They will help you remember that you are still the same person inside, with the same loves that you had before your injury. No one and no injury can take that away from you.

<u>Don't expect to be "who you used to be" right away.</u>

Brain injury is a life-altering event. Try to think in terms of healing and rebuilding who you are. It takes time. Many things about you have probably changed. This is not always a bad thing. Some survivors find they have become more patient and understanding.

<u>Try email and phone calls.</u>

You'll know when you are ready to start reaching out. Email and phone calls are easier to control and less threatening.

<u>Try a support group for brain injury survivors.</u>

Pick the time when you feel ready for a group of people with similar experiences. You may need to try more than one group to find a good "fit" for you.

<u>Try to connect with one of the support group members outside the group.</u>

Someone who has similar issues can be the best support and feel the least threatening.

<u>Consider trying passive activities first.</u>

This might be a relatively quiet activity where you don't need to interact much, where you can just listen and watch, like a movie, attending a lecture, a stage play or a concert. Bookstores frequently offer free lectures by local and popular authors. (Sit where you can gracefully escape if need be.)

<u>Attend events that interest you.</u>

You will enjoy the event and you will have something in common to chat with the others about.

Helpful Strategies: Set Yourself Up to Succeed!

- ❏ Limit your exposure to crowds and confusion. Plan to stay a short time or have a quiet place to retreat to when you start to feel overwhelmed.
- ❏ Go to restaurants before 5:00 to avoid the crowds - and save some money!
- ❏ Buy a wallet size tip card with a chart for tips and taxes. (often available at card stores) or let someone else figure it out.
- ❏ Carry your earplugs with you at all times if noise is a problem for you.
- ❏ Wear a cap or visor or carry your sunglasses with you at all times if bright lights or fluorescent lights are a problem for you.
- ❏ Make a plan for social activities. Make a few notes to take with you. If you forget, go to a private place and review them, like the bathroom or your car.
    - ○ Think about where you are going and why?
    - ○ Who will likely be there?
    - ○ What are their interests?
    - ○ What are some possible questions you might ask?
- ❏ Prepare for family gatherings. Review photo albums or ask a family member to help refresh your memory about relatives **before** the event.
- ❏ Try to hold conversations in a quiet place. Ask people to speak one at a time, so you can hear them. When that is not possible, just try to listen and smile!
- ❏ If you find questions about yourself at social events overwhelming, try answering briefly and then turn the question around, asking the same question of the other person. Sometimes you can find a small way to help out, like passing something out, to avoid long conversations. Taking photographs at the event is another way to limit interaction.
- ❏ Plan an easy day before a big event and "down time" the day after. Sometimes it may not be until you get home that you realize how draining the occasion was.

Practice Good Listening Skills

"To be truly with people in conversation, I think of myself, of my whole body, as an ear."

— Maya Angelou

❏ Let it be OK not to say everything you think of, forget or don't have time to say. I think talking is overrated but it can be a hard habit to break. Don't we all appreciate a good listener?

❏ Good communicators listen more than they talk. Make a decision to listen; it is not a natural reflex.

❏ Listen for both the actual words and the feelings behind the words, how the words are spoken; non-verbal, facial and body gestures, posture and eye contact.

❏ Listening and hearing are different things. Listening is paying attention to what you hear.

❏ Don't let yourself be distracted by your cell phone or other electronic devices.

❏ Imagine the speaker in the spotlight and try to focus only on him or her.

❏ Comment on what you think a person is saying and ask if you understood correctly.

❏ Be aware of "tuning out" – daydreaming, being on automatic pilot, fidgeting, arms crossed, interrupting and finishing sentences.

❏ If you tend to want to interrupt because you're afraid you will lose your thought; try using a notepad, when possible, to write down key words that you can use as memory joggers later, when it is your turn to speak

❏ If you tend to ramble on, as you try to organize your thoughts:
   ○ Make a list of talking points before you make a call and leave space to make notes about the response.
   ○ When you are speaking directly to a person or a group, watch for attentiveness in others. Are they still making eye contact with you? If not, it's your cue to finish talking. If a family member is with you, ask them to give you a subtle signal when they notice you are rambling.

Phone Skills: Prepare for the conversation:

❏ Create an environment conducive to listening and processing information - minimize distractions and interruptions:

  ○ Make calls when you have the house to yourself or close the door to the room and let others know you need quiet.

  ○ Take the dog out before you begin.

  ○ Turn off the TV.

  ○ Get into a comfortable position.

  ○ Do you need to put a headset on?

  ○ Sit where you can see a clock or set a timer.

  ○ Don't answer "call waiting" unless it is absolutely necessary.

❏ For personal calls, review any notes you made before you begin.

❏ For business calls, have a pencil, your Telephone Log (sample in Chapter 4 on Improving Memory) and your folder with any other pertinent information in front of you before you begin.

❏ Review your goal for this phone call:

  ○ Do you want it to be brief?

  ○ Do you need to give specific information?

  ○ Do you need to get specific information?

  ○ Would it help to script questions before the call?

❏ Suggestions for keeping personal calls short:

  ○ "I only have a couple of minutes but I wanted to talk to you."

  ○ "I only have until about ____ o'clock but I wanted to talk with you"

  ○ "I have to leave in a few minutes but I'm glad you called."

❏ Suggestions for sustaining a conversation:

  ○ "Tell me what you've been up to lately?"

  ○ "So update me on your family."

  ○ "Tell me about your plans for the _____"

❏ Suggestions for ending a call:

  ○ "It has been good to talk to you. I'm sorry, I have to go."

  ○ "Oops, it's almost __(time)__, I have to go."

  ○ "I'm getting too tired to be a good listener. I need to go."

  ○ "I'm sorry, I really can't talk now. When is a good time to call you back?"

❏ Practice "active listening", focusing on what is being said.

❏ Consider prepaid long distance phone cards to help control costs.

<u>Relationship building blocks:</u> to help build social skills.

- ❏ Get along with family and people at rehabilitation first.
- ❏ Can you put someone else at ease?
- ❏ Can you keep a conversation going for 10 minutes?
- ❏ Is there give and take in the conversation, talking and *listening*?
- ❏ Prepare and practice questions.

<u>Components to consider in relationships,</u> to help you troubleshoot any difficulties you are having with relationships.

- ❏ What do you have to offer?
- ❏ What are you looking for?
- ❏ Are you demonstrating the above?
- ❏ Relationships are hard for *everyone* and ongoing.
- ❏ TV and Internet are NOT reality.

<u>Tips for building rewarding friendships:</u>

- ❏ Be positive, and upbeat, smiles are catchy.
- ❏ Be sure you balance talking and listening.
- ❏ Respect and accept different opinions.
- ❏ Be honest and reliable.
- ❏ Talk about others in a positive way.

"The biggest roadblock to independent living in society is not the physical deficits or even the cognitive problems involved in brain injury. It's behavior with a capital B. The welcome mat will not be put out for you if you're argumentative, nasty, bossy and difficult to deal with."

— Richard Senelick, M.D. and Karla Doherty
Living with Brain Injury

Dealing with new situations can be scary and intimidating at first but it will get easier. Healing and time will bring you more comfort with the "new you". Many skills can improve. Your tolerance for sounds, lights and confusion will likely moderate in time. You will get to know your usual problem areas and be able to strategize around them.

Remember to reward yourself for situations handled well. Trying something new requires courage! Give yourself a pat on the back and spend time doing something you really love to do. Acknowledging successes helps build self-confidence!

Conversation Evaluator
For the SPEAKER

As a SPEAKER, did you:

	Yes	Sometimes	No
Face your listener?	____	____	____
Keep eye contact?	____	____	____
Use appropriate expression?	____	____	____
Watch for listener reaction?	____	____	____
Answer your listener's questions?	____	____	____
Stay on topic?	____	____	____
Give clear information?	____	____	____
Use appropriate volume?	____	____	____
Enjoy having the conversation?	____	____	____
Did you take turns being the SPEAKER and the LISTENER?	____	____	____

Conversation Evaluator

For the LISTENER

As a LISTENER, did you:

	Yes	Sometimes	No
Face your speaker?	_____	_____	_____
Keep eye contact?	_____	_____	_____
Listen for the words and the feelings?	_____	_____	_____
Avoid interrupting?	_____	_____	_____
Comment on what the person said?	_____	_____	_____
Ask appropriate questions?	_____	_____	_____
Stay focused and not "tune out"?	_____	_____	_____
Enjoy having the conversation?	_____	_____	_____
Enjoy having the conversation?	_____	_____	_____
Did you take turns being the LISTENER and the SPEAKER?	_____	_____	_____

Note: It will probably be helpful to look at this before a social situation for tips to keep in mind, as well as afterwards, to evaluate.

Creative Problem-Solving Worksheet Example

1. Identify the problem - what is the issue?

Large family gatherings! I can't remember who people are or what to say to them. I get tired and overwhelmed. I get upset and want to go home.

2. Focus your energies in a positive direction.

What can I do to learn from this?

Find a way to remember who people are and how not to get so tired.

3. Think of several solutions:

Possible Solution #1

Review family photos before family events to help me remember who's who.

Possible Solution #2

Shorten the visit so I don't get overtired and cranky.

Possible Solution #3

Take my earplugs with me and find a quiet place if I start getting a headache or feeling overwhelmed.

Best Solution

Using all strategies above!

4. Put your solutions into practice.

Looked at family album with sister before the wedding to refresh my memory. Took earplugs. Talked to sister ahead of time about possibly needing to leave early.

5. Review.

What worked?

Reviewing family photos a huge help! Put earplugs in when the band started. Left after dessert. I didn't get cranky!

What didn't work?

I still forgot names and who was who, I asked a lot of questions. I felt stupid. Sometimes people seemed a little irritated.

What will I try next time?

Taking some photos with me with some notes on the backs so I can sneak a peek to help me remember. Let it be OK not to remember; listen more.

Creative Problem-Solving Worksheet

1. Identify the problem - what is the issue?

2. Focus your energies in a positive direction.
    What can I learn from this?

3. Think of several solutions:
    Possible Solution #1

    Possible Solution #2

    Possible Solution #3

    Best Solution

4. Put your solutions into practice.
    Try out your best possible solution

5. Review.
    What worked?

    What didn't work?

    What will I try next time?

Listen

When I ask you to listen to me,
And you start giving me advice,
You have not done what I asked.

When I ask you to listen to me,
And you begin to tell me why I shouldn't feel that way,
You are trampling on my feelings.

When I ask you to listen to me,
And you feel you have to do something to solve my problems,
You have failed me, strange as that may seem.

Listen: All that I ask is that you listen,
Not talk or do – just hear me.

When you do something for me
That I need to do for myself,
You contribute to my fear and feelings of inadequacy.

But when you accept as a simple fact
That I do feel what I feel, no matter how irrational,
Then I can quit trying to convince you
And go about the business
Of understanding what's behind my feelings.

So, please listen and just hear me
And if you want to talk,
Wait a minute for your turn – and I'll listen to you.

— Author unknown

The Four Agreements

Be Impeccable With Your Word

Speak with integrity. Say only what you mean.
Avoid using the word to speak against yourself
or to gossip about others. Use the power of your
word in the direction of truth and love.

Don't Take Anything Personally

Nothing others do is because of you. What others say
and do is a projection of their own reality, their own dream.
When you are immune to the opinions and actions of others,
you won't be the victim of needless suffering.

Don't Make Assumptions

Find the courage to ask questions and to express
what you really want. Communicate with others
as clearly as you can to avoid misunderstandings,
sadness, and drama. With just this one agreement,
you can completely transform your life.

Always Do Your Best

Your best is going to change from moment to moment;
it will be different when you are healthy as opposed to sick.
Under any circumstance, simply do your best,
and you will avoid self-judgment, self-abuse, and regret.

— Don Miguel Ruiz

A Complex and Dangerous Task

Strategies for Driving and Directions

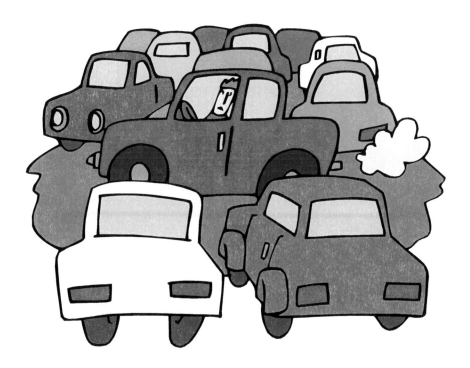

A Complex and Dangerous Task

Strategies for Driving and Directions

*"Don't let your past dictate who you are
but let it be a part of who you will become."*

— Dear Abby

Driving represents independence. It is something we usually take for granted. It is natural to want to return to driving after a brain injury. However, driving is the most dangerous thing we do in our every day lives, the ultimate multi-tasking experience! Your safety as well as the safety of others is at stake.

Driving requires many physical and mental abilities; memory, visual skills, processing speed, judgment and decision-making skills. Check with your local Registry of Motor Vehicles before you return to driving; the laws and regulations vary from state to state. Driving evaluations and training are available through rehabilitation programs. A driving evaluation is a crucial step in determining a person's ability to drive after a brain injury, for the survivor and for family members.

Even if you feel physically and mentally ready, it still might not be a good idea for you to drive a car for a while. Test yourself, carefully and gradually. Try driving a short distance in good weather and when the traffic is light, perhaps in a vacant parking lot or in your neighborhood. Ask yourself how you might react if you were suddenly cut-off in traffic by a teenager or a sports car.

**The Suggestions In This Chapter Assume
You Are "Safe To Drive".**

Safe Driving Tips

Remember: 1 Alcoholic drink = 3 alcoholic drinks for a brain injury survivor.

Due to the changes in your brain chemistry, the effects of alcohol are magnified. The side effects of some medications (like drowsiness), can be multiplied by alcoholic drinks.

Limit driving time to 20 minutes at first, until your stamina increases.

Avoid driving during peak traffic times.

Avoid highway driving in the beginning.

It requires faster processing and a sense of direction to determine the correct exit: Do I get off the highway at Exit 4 North or Exit 4 South?

Be extra cautious about driving at night.

Brain injury can cause visual changes that you might not be aware of. For example sensitivity to lights.

Try polarized sunglasses for driving glare.

Try yellow tinted glasses for night driving.

Travel the same basic routes when possible.

Repetition aids memory and it will help to minimize confusion and anxiety. You will learn shortcuts in time.

Use extra caution:

❏ When turning left against oncoming traffic
❏ When pedestrians and bicyclists are present
❏ Around construction sites and detours

Limit distractions.

Travel when you're rested and alert, the traffic is light and the weather is good as much as possible and especially when you are starting to drive again after your injury.

❏ Place your cell phone in the glove compartment or on back seat or out of reach so you won't be tempted to answer it while you are driving. **Know the laws regarding cell phone use and driving in your state.**

❏ Fasten your seatbelt.

❏ Set the controls for the lights, wipers, heater, air conditioner, radio, etc. **before** you begin to drive.

❑ Resist the temptation to eat or drink while driving.

❑ If the radio is distracting or making you feel anxious, turn it off or try playing a tape/CD with some soft instrumental music instead.

❑ Explain to passengers that you have trouble driving and talking at the same time. You might ask for their help reading street signs and finding landmarks. Children like to help this way too.

Plan extra time.

This will help you with any and all other strategies you need to use. Plan at least <u>double</u> the travel time you used to.

❑ To minimize stress and anxiety.

❑ To allow for traffic and wrong turns.

❑ To pull over and "decompress" if you get confused or overwhelmed. Take some slow deep breaths, close your eyes for a few moments, drink some water.

❑ To consult your directions or a map or call for assistance.

❑ To find a parking space.

❑ To find the office, use the restroom and collect yourself before the appointment.

For longer trips

Take a copilot with you, if possible; for support, to help read signs and directions, or to take over when you get tired.

For appointments

Take the office phone number or the appointment card with you, in case you need help with directions or you get delayed.

Park in the same general area of the parking lot each time you go somewhere.

The routine will help you remember where your car is!

Park so you can **Head Out** of a parking space.

Do this, when possible, instead of backing out. You'll have much better visibility.

Do you find yourself not remembering how you got somewhere?

You are probably tired, stressed and/or distracted. You are driving on "automatic pilot" and not focused on your driving so things aren't registering in your brain as you do them. Try to eliminate distractions; turn off the radio, pull over and collect yourself; then concentrate on driving. Try talking to yourself about where you are going and the landmarks you are passing.

<u>Trouble figuring out how to get somewhere?</u>

You probably have trouble with "spatial relationships". You will need to do some planning before you go somewhere; get directions, use maps and/or take a dry run. Here are some strategies I use:

1. Using Directions:

   ❏ Study ahead of time and check with a map.
   ❏ Ask for landmarks, to give you visual cues.
   ❏ Print directions in a large font for easier reading while driving.
   ❏ Write or print out directions <u>both ways</u> – in reverse for your return trip.
   ❏ Double check Internet directions with a map, they can be confusing, like when they use different names for streets.
   ❏ Keep maps in your car to refer to if necessary.

2. Using Internet directions and navigation or "global positioning systems" (GPS) can be a godsend in unfamiliar territory but they have their drawbacks:

   ❏ They take some getting used to.
   ❏ Don't expect them to be 100% accurate.
   ❏ They may take you the "shortest route" by using back roads, making it easy to get "turned around" and harder to learn your way.
   ❏ You may not always be able to access satellite reception.

   <u>Recommendations:</u>

   ❏ Be sure to use a GPS that speaks street names so you don't have to look at it while you are driving.
   ❏ Practice using your GPS as a passenger and then as a driver, before you depend on it in unfamiliar territory.
   ❏ Program your GPS before you leave the house, to be sure you'll have the addresses you need.
   ❏ Use your GPS and Internet directions in conjunction with the other strategies that you find helpful when following directions.

3. Taking a dry run in the car is especially helpful for new locations and stressful appointments. Take a practice trip at low stress/low traffic times like a Sunday afternoon before the appointment. You may want to take two dry runs; one as the copilot and one as the driver.

<u>Label and save directions and phone numbers for future use.</u>

Designate a section in your planner for them. If you do not carry a planner you can use an envelope or plastic sheet saver and keep it in the glove compartment of your car.

<u>Using a compass may help you with directions.</u>

You can purchase a portable one to mount on your dashboard if your car doesn't come equipped with one.

If you are starting to feel overwhelmed

When you are stopped in traffic or at a red light:

- ❏ Try slow deep breathing, expanding and contracting your stomach, counting to seven with each inhale and exhale.

- ❏ Try involving another sense by eating a strong flavored piece of candy or gum.

- ❏ Try squeezing the steering wheel and counting to 10.

If you continue to feel overwhelmed

Stop at the nearest parking lot or rest area and take a break.
Do some stretching or walk around a little, eat a snack, take a short nap.

You are most likely to feel drowsy between lunch and dinner.

This is due to your blood sugar level dropping. Having a snack, drinking some coffee or water can help.

Don't wait too long to ask for help.

Fatigue and anxiety inhibit cognition. If you ask for directions, repeat them back to check for accuracy. Write them down when possible.

Calls to 911 are FREE.

You can carry an old cell phone and charger, without an active service provider, for emergency calls. 911 Calls go to the State Police. You will need to <u>know your location</u> when you call.

Driving is a tiring, complex task. As you heal physically you will feel more capable.

Anything you do that improves your cognition will also help your driving skills. Suggestions are crossword puzzles, playing cards or board games like Scrabble. Jigsaw puzzles, reading, learning something new and exercising can all help your cognition and reaction times.

Keep in mind that the cost of operating a car for one year is substantial. Thousands of dollars, *without a car loan.* That is a lot of money you can use for public transportation or to pay people to give you a ride.

Safe Driver Checklist

❏ Can you read road signs clearly and understand what they indicate?

❏ Do you have difficulty seeing clearly at dusk and in the dark?

❏ Do headlights from other vehicles interfere with your vision?

❏ Do you forget the basics, such as wearing your seatbelt, putting on your headlights or putting on the windshield wipers in the rain?

❏ Do you have trouble keeping up with the posted speed limit?

❏ Do passing vehicles, trucks and motorcycles, frighten you?

❏ Are your reflexes and reaction time quick enough to be able to respond to other drivers who may be driving erratically, for example stopping short in front of you?

❏ Do you have difficulties following detours or seeing a police officer directing traffic?

❏ Do you often find yourself lost on what were once familiar roads?

❏ Do you have trouble figuring out what to do at intersections, for example when it is safe to proceed?

❏ Do you get drowsy, have difficulty concentrating or frequently become overwhelmed and need to pull over to take a break, while you are driving?

❏ Have your family or friends told you that you shouldn't be driving?

If you find yourself answering yes to many of these questions, consider driving less or not at all, at least for the time being. Taking a driver training course may help you restore your skills and confidence.

Winter Driving Tips

Driving in winter is probably the most difficult and hazardous of driving conditions. Motor vehicles handle much differently on snow and ice than they do on dry pavement. I avoid driving in stormy weather whenever possible, keeping the weather forecast in mind when I plan my week.

<u>General tips for winter driving:</u>

- ❏ Make sure your windshield wipers and defroster are in good condition. Fill your windshield washer reservoir with a cleaning solution that will not freeze.

- ❏ Keep your fuel tank at least half full in case you get stuck in traffic and to prevent the fuel line from freezing.

- ❏ Before driving, remove ice and snow from your vehicle. Clear all of the windows, lights and the roof of the vehicle.

- ❏ If it is snowing, start slowly. Test your brakes by tapping them gently to see how much traction your tires have.

- ❏ Reduce your speed according to road conditions. Drive cautiously and accelerate gently.

- ❏ Increase the space between your vehicle and others. You need more distance to stop safely on slippery roads.

- ❏ Never brake hard on icy roads; you will lose steering control. If you do skid, remember to turn into the direction of the skid.

- ❏ Bridges and highway overpasses tend to freeze before the rest of the road and can be unexpectedly slippery.

- ❏ Keep a blanket, flashlight and a small shovel in your trunk.

- ❏ If you get stuck in your car in the snow, make sure your exhaust pipe is cleared of snow.

Yes, You Can!

Suggestions for Rebuilding Skills and a Life After Brain Injury

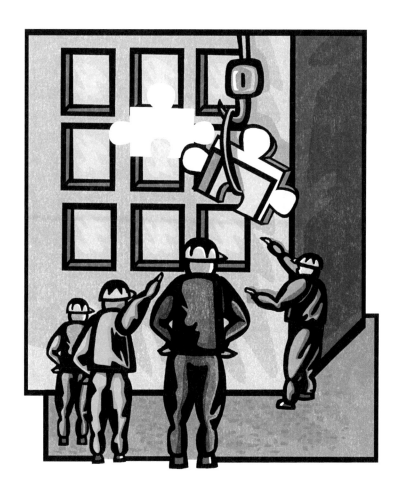

Yes, You Can!

Suggestions for Rebuilding Skills and a Life After Brain Injury

*"The most satisfying moments come when we
work through our biggest challenges."*

— Tedy Bruschi, Stroke Survivor

Finally, emerging science is catching up with what we survivors have known for years - that the brain can heal and that we can regain and rebuild skills! With advancements in imagery technology, our knowledge base of how the brain functions and can change is rapidly increasing. The evidence is mounting regarding the positive effects of stimuli like diet, exercise, music, art, continued learning and challenging the brain!

"Scientists used to think that the adult brain was hard-wired and unchangeable, making learning and responding to new experiences more difficult. We now know that the brain has a lifelong capacity to change in both structure and function, a capability called neuroplasticity. The brain can adapt and heal itself after injury, restructure neuronal networks in response to new knowledge and new demands, and even generate new cells. And evidence suggests it's possible to promote this adaptability through healthy lifestyle choices."

— "Mind, Mood and Memory" July 2009
Massachusetts General Hospital

Rehabilitation, even from a "mild" brain injury (as if there is any such thing!) typically continues long after rehabilitation services are no longer available to brain injury survivors, often due to insurance and financial limitations. The good news is that there are many things we can do ourselves! To find those building blocks, I suggest beginning with something that interests you; something you've wished you had more time for, something you always wanted to do, something you are passionate about. Think about what you liked to do in your free time, as a child and before your injury, any hobbies you enjoyed. These are clues to your passions. Your enthusiasm and passion will help to give you the extra motivation and energy necessary for figuring out how to do it now.

Through practice and persistence, improvements can be truly amazing! This chapter contains some suggestions to help you with the rebuilding process by:

❏ Managing Your Stress
❏ Exercise
❏ Getting Involved in the Arts
❏ Working with Music

❏ Doing a PhotoVoice Project
❏ Playing "Brain Games"
❏ Other Possibilities
❏ Volunteering

Managing Your Stress

Practice breathing from your diaphragm and meditation, every day! They are the body's natural, built-in, antidotes to stress. Stress inhibits learning. Meditation is the only way I found to give my brain a rest, as if it were in a cast. Meditation is the only way I found to shut off the never ending tape of "musts" and "shoulds" in my mind. Meditation is the only way I found to re-boot when it feels like there is a logjam in my brain.

Please refer to the suggestions in Chapter 2 on managing stress and overload, and find a stress management tool that works for you.

Exercise

There is a growing body of research demonstrating that regular aerobic exercise, even brisk walking, boosts brainpower by stimulating neurogenesis, the formation of new brain cells (neurons). Exercise also strengthens connections between those cells. Researchers have found the areas of the brain that are stimulated through exercise are associated with memory and learning!

Exercise doesn't have to be complicated. Any movement is exercise. You can even exercise while seated in a chair or beside a chair to help you with balance. The goal is to get your heart beating faster than it normally does and to exercise regularly.

If you have difficulties with balance, please consult a physical therapist. If physical therapy doesn't help, you may need to consult a visual therapist for vestibular therapy. Balance difficulties can be caused by problems with your vision and receptors in the inner ear, the vestibular system.

Exercise has many benefits:

❏ Exercise gets your blood flowing and increases oxygen to your brain.

❏ Exercise supports the formation of new brain cells.

❏ Exercise changes tension in your body and carrying tension can be very tiring.

❏ Exercise raises endorphins - those "feel good" chemicals.

❏ Exercise helps to normalize melatonin production in your brain and enhance your sleep cycle. However, avoid exercising two hours before bedtime.

❏ A 10-minute walk, just 10 minutes, gives you more of an energy boost than a candy bar!

❏ Exercise increases metabolism and helps keep weight down.

Try doing your daily activities in reverse!

Activities involving the use of right and left help build cross-connections in your brain and can help you with balance, problem solving and organization skills!

For example:

- ❏ When you are getting dressed and putting on your pants, if you usually put the right leg on first, instead try putting the left leg on first. Try putting your left sleeve on first, your left sock and shoe first.

- ❏ If you are right handed, try drinking with your left hand. Try eating with your left hand.

- ❏ Try playing a game with your left hand. It is harder than you think!

Try different kinds of exercise.

Try something different. Try dance – any kind of dance, your own kind of dancing to music in the privacy of your home! Try yoga, Tai Chi, water therapy. Any activity that you enjoy, even while seated, that gets your heart beating faster is good for your body and your brain. Whatever you do, experiment and have fun!

The structure of a regular class can be helpful.

Check out programs sponsored by local schools and hospitals, they are usually inexpensive. Check out recreation programs for people with disabilities. You won't believe the kinds of adaptive equipment available

Play!

Don't underestimate the power of play. You are using multiple skills by participating in almost any activity. Recreational activities provide a vehicle for building social skills as well as cognitive skills - while having some fun at the same time! Think of simple activities you enjoyed as a child. If you have children, play with them. When you are engaged in something you enjoy, you feel energized. Play supports learning, memory and well-being. Play is a natural stress reducer.

Getting Involved in the Arts

Participate in art therapy if you can. Take an art class or work on your own. Learn something new or go back to something you used to do. Work in any medium that interests you – drama, painting, music, drumming, clay, photography, knitting, scrap booking. Working with art helps to process emotions and build skills, particularly organizational skills. It can be especially helpful if you're more of a "hands-on" learner.

Working With Music

See "The Power of Music" at the end of Chapter 4.

Doing a PhotoVoice Project

Doing a PhotoVoice Project can be an extraordinary vehicle for processing the emotions associated with healing from a brain injury, while providing a variety of opportunities for skill building and raising brain injury awareness. A PhotoVoice Project Guide is provided at the end of this workbook. You may also be able to view examples of PhotoVoice Projects by brain injury survivors on www.biama.org and www.brainline.org

Playing "Brain Games"

Play any game that interests and challenges you – card games, board games, dominoes, jigsaw puzzles, crossword puzzles. The challenge is the key to help your brain.

Scrabble

Two-letter words are OK!

Tribond

You can play this as a board game with others or you can use the cards like flash cards and play by yourself.

Jigsaw puzzles

Start small. There is nothing wrong with a 10-piece jigsaw puzzle! Make room for it on a table that you pass by frequently. Encourage others to participate! Work on jigsaw puzzle maps of the United States and the world to help you with your geography.

Working with crossword puzzles

Clip crossword puzzles from the newspaper and make 3 copies or buy 3 copies of an easy crossword puzzle book. Work in pencil and eraser, a big frustration saver!

- ❏ Work on copy 1 using the solution page as often as you like.
  (This is not cheating!)

- ❏ Wait a day and work on copy 2, trying to recall the answers from the previous day. Feel free to refer to the solution page.

- ❏ Wait a day and work on copy 3. Can you see improvement?

Play with other brain injury survivors, children or an elderly person.

It may be the least intimidating way to start, you will all benefit.

Teach a friend to play your favorite game!

Refer to Hoyle's Rules of Games to refresh your memory about rules for games.

"Challenging your brain creates new neural pathways. Just like you challenge a muscle to grow it, well, the brain gets new connections. Want to keep your brain young? Exercise it. Try learning to play a musical instrument, doing crossword puzzles, learning a language – even playing computer games. ***The data now indicate than an hour of games for 40 weeks can make your brain equivalent, your brain's real age, to 10 years younger." !!!***

— Dr. Michael F. Roizen and Dr. Mehmet Oz
You: The Owner's Manual

Other Possiblities

Use workbooks meant for children.

Work in pencil and eraser. Try not to feel insulted by working at such a low skill level at first. Try to think of it as creating building blocks for healing and rehabilitating your brain. Sometimes you have to take a step backwards, in order to be able to take a step forward.

Use flashcards.

There are all types of flash cards for math and vocabulary. If you are having trouble remembering family members, you can make your own flashcards using their photos and writing information about them on the back.

Use the newspaper.

- ❏ Memorize one headline, turn it over, see if you can remember it to say it or write it down.
- ❏ Read an article in a magazine or the newspaper; retell it in your own words or write a summary.

Challenge yourself to think of or write down as many words as you can think of for each letter of the alphabet.

How many words can you think of that start with the letter A. . .B. . .C. . . This is a good travel game - for passengers!

Memorize favorite poems or songs or dance steps.

Learn to identify birds, flowers, leaves, rocks.

Do whatever interests you! I liked geology so in taking my son to rock and mineral shows, I started learning and re-learning the names of the rocks. It felt really good to know something and I was able to help my son learn as well!

Learn or restore typing skills.

Use a typing tutorial on the computer.

Learn or restore music skills.

Start with beginners books and re-teach yourself. Write in the names of the notes below the notes.

Take an adult education class.

Pick something that you want to learn or re-learn, anything that interests you! These classes are low cost and low stress, there are no grades to worry about!

Build your cooking skills!

Try a new cookbook, try new recipes! Make a booklet of your favorite recipes.

Join a book discussion group.

If you can't find one to join, start one with other brain injury survivors.

Take a virtual trip.

Pick a place you've always wanted to go. Learn all about it! Listen to the music. Cook some recipes typical of the location. Take a class about it. Learn the language.

Do what you enjoy!

Doing what you enjoy is more important than the specific activity. Many survivors find that they are more creative after their injury.

Volunteer

Volunteer work can be a low risk way to take the next step to test and brush up on skills in the world of work. It is a commitment and there are expectations but you don't have the threat of losing a paycheck if it doesn't work out. People tend to be very appreciative of volunteers – and why not – they are getting your services for free! Feeling appreciated is a huge self-confidence builder.

Think about what interests you, try to find a volunteer opportunity where they are used to having volunteers and may have some training. If something doesn't work out, learn from it and try something else. (See Creative Problem Solving Worksheet in Chapter 13)

When you are learning something new, try to stick with one teacher or support person. Try to find a person who is patient and good at explaining things step by step. Different people have different ways of doing things and it can become confusing if you are working with more than one person.

<u>Possibilities for volunteer work:</u>

- ❏ Assume a small responsibility within a group you already belong to.
- ❏ Help out with any cause that is dear to your heart.
- ❏ Read to children – in your family, local nursery school, library.
- ❏ Assist the elderly – local senior center, nursing home, neighbor.
- ❏ Help at your child's school.
- ❏ Help out at your local library.
- ❏ ESL Teacher (English as a Second Language) – check with your local library for programs.
- ❏ Red Cross and other non-profit organization.
- ❏ Start a brain injury support group!
- ❏ Volunteer for the Brain Injury Association in your state.

Remember to start small; even a couple of hours, one morning a week, is a good start! Set yourself up to succeed. It will feel much better to be able to add more hours than it will feel if you get tired from trying to do too much and have to back down or quit.

The Rehabilitation Process

I see the process of rehabilitation after a brain injury as a series of "building blocks" that build on the strategies you learn from one step to the next. You will need to make adjustments in how much you can do from time to time as life presents other challenges. When you feel you are comfortable handling what you are doing consistently for several months and maybe even starting to get bored, then you are ready to move on to the next step! The steps will vary depending on your situation. The basic building blocks for me were:

- ❏ Taking care of yourself; personal hygiene, getting dressed appropriately, attending medical appointments
- ❏ Managing home and family;preparing meals, doing laundry, assisting with children's schoolwork, paying bills
- ❏ Managing tasks in the community like shopping and errands, children's school activities, church
- ❏ Engaging in a hobby or activity you are passionate about
- ❏ Volunteer work
- ❏ Meaningful (paid or unpaid) work

				Volunteer/Work
			Hobby	Hobby
		Community	Community	Community
	Home & Family	Home & Family	Home & Family	Home & Family
Self Care	Self Care	Self Care	Self Care	Self Care

I think the ultimate challenge for brain injury survivors, as they heal and recreate their lives, is to find a way to feel useful again. Like other people, we want to feel like our lives have value and purpose. This may involve a realignment of values and priorities, gained from the perspective of surviving a traumatic event. The brain injury experience has a way of throwing you into a "self-crisis" along with a lot of the other life-crises. As a result, you may define what is significant, useful and valuable differently now than you did before your injury.

We were all unique individuals before our injuries and the brain injury doesn't change that. Only you can discover and travel the path in this new chapter of your life. It won't be easy and you will need a lot of courage but it is possible to recreate a meaningful life. It is my hope that the suggestions in this guide will make your journey a little easier and give you hope that you can heal and improve your life after a brain injury.

"What would you attempt if you knew you would not fail?"

— Unknown

Believe in Yourself!

Celebrate Your Successes!

You Can Improve!

Assets and Strengths

Complete the following questions with the first thing that comes to mind. Keep your answers short and simple. If you are stumped by a question, move on. It is not necessary to answer them all. Have fun with it!

1. My favorite thing to do with my free time is ...

2. My friends would describe me as a person who is ...

3. Something that I find very beautiful is ...

4. Something that I really enjoy doing is ...

5. One of the things people like about me is that I am ...

6. Three words I would use to describe myself are ...

7. Three things I do well are ...

8. A place that I really enjoy being is ... because ...

9. If I were to receive an award, it would be for ...

10. A project or undertaking that I have been most proud of is ...

11. I am really inspired by ...

12. With age I have developed my ability to ...

13. One of the things I enjoy spending time thinking about is ...

14. One of the things I enjoy learning about is ...

15. My creativity is expressed through my ...

16. Something that I am passionate about is ...

17. Something that I would like to be remembered for in my life is ...

These answers are the clues to your passions, your strengths and your healing path.

The things you love are your gifts. These are the things the brain injury could not take away from you.

Star Qualities

A. Name 3 people you admire, respect or think highly of.

B. List 2 qualities about each person listed.

Why do you admire, respect or think highly of them?

Person	Qualities

C. Copy the qualities you listed above into the star below.

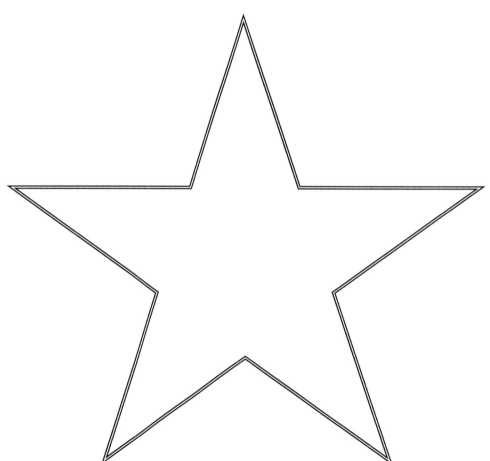

**The qualities that you listed and copied into the star are
YOUR STAR QUALITIES!**

It is said that you admire characteristics in others because you have them or are developing them in yourself. Give it some thought and see if it feels true to you.

Making Changes

According to psychologists, self-evaluation happens every 5-10 years and is a normal part of lifelong growth. Traumatic experiences intensify these transitions and as a result, priorities, needs and lifestyles may change. Here are three steps to help you transition and move ahead and continue healing:

1. Know yourself and define your purpose.

This is your reason for being, why you get up each day. It may help to think about:

- ❏ Three accomplishments that make you feel great – in any area, leisure, social, work, church, civic.
- ❏ Activities that you loved as a child
- ❏ What would you do if it were impossible for you to fail?
- ❏ How would you make the world better?
- ❏ When does your body feel most alive?

2. Brainstorm options with someone who knows you well.

Someone close to you often recognizes things you don't. To explore further you may want to take a class or do some volunteer work, interview friends about their jobs.

3. Outline your goal, strategies and timeline.

Take small steps. Your first step may be to set aside time on a regular basis to work towards your goal. Visualize yourself living your goal. Modify your goal as needed. View setbacks as "learning experiences". Avoid "I can't", instead, think, "How?"

4. What is the next step for you?

"You are braver than you believe, and stronger than you seem, and smarter than you think."

— Christopher Robin, Winnie the Pooh's friend

The Tao Of Success

"Nothing in the world can take the place of Persistence.

Talent will not; nothing is more commonplace than unsuccessful men with talent.

Genius will not; unrewarded genius is almost a proverb.

Education alone will not; the world is full of educated derelicts.

Persistence and Determination alone are omnipotent."

— Calvin Coolidge

Tools

PhotoVoice Project Guide

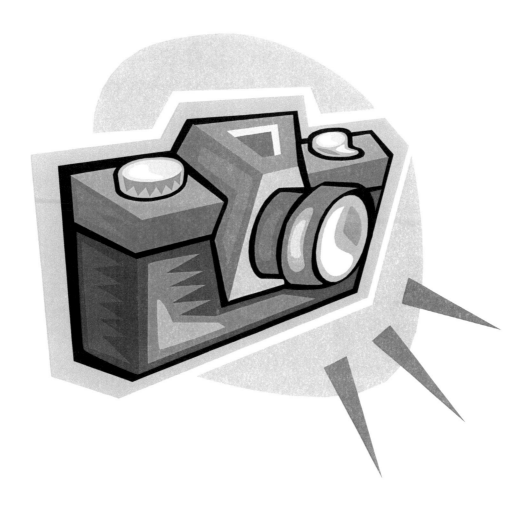

Introduction to PhotoVoice

What is PhotoVoice?

PhotoVoice is a process by which people can represent their lives, points of view and experience, using pictures and narratives.

PhotoVoice was developed by Caroline Wang in the early 1990s as a method for raising awareness about rural development issues and helping women in rural communities in China to become part of the policy making process, to give them a "voice".

PhotoVoice is "inside out" photojournalism. Instead of illustrating a story with photos, the subjects themselves take the photographs that are meaningful to them and then explain their significance with narratives. PhotoVoice is not about the quality of the photographs taken.

PhotoVoice is a very flexible process; it has been done in different ways and with different populations, around the world.

PhotoVoice Projects provide an opportunity for survivors to:
- ❏ Reflect on living with brain injury
- ❏ Use their brain in new ways and employ a variety of skills
- ❏ Raise awareness about brain injury
- ❏ Help health care providers understand ways to support healing from a brain injury

How did the Brain Injury Survivor Support Group in Framingham, MA get involved with PhotoVoice?

The Framingham group had the good fortune to discover PhotoVoice through Laura Lorenz, PhD, a health policy researcher and former photojournalist who had used PhotoVoice with township youth in South Africa and Girls Inc. in the United States. She also used it as a pilot study for her doctoral research with a member of our support group and with brain injury survivors through Spaulding Rehabilitation Hospital in Boston.

What is special about doing a PhotoVoice Project?

The Framingham PhotoVoice Project members found the project to be much more than we ever expected. When you stop to think about it, you are using many, many skills to do a PhotoVoice Project; large and fine motor skills, visual skills, a variety of language skills, organizational and problem solving skills. You are also being creative and reflecting on your experience as a brain injury survivor. The more involved you become with the project, the more you will gain from the process. The Framingham group found PhotoVoice to be a rehabilitation tool, a vehicle that promoted the healing process. It helped participants move on. It changed lives.

<u>How do PhotoVoice Projects help raise awareness about brain injury?</u>

When you do a PhotoVoice Project you are creating something concrete that you can share with others. You can use the notebooks you create to help family, friends and health care professionals better understand your brain injury. As an option you may also want to create a public exhibit of your photos and narratives. Three years later, the Framingham PhotoVoice Project group continues to use their project to help raise awareness about brain injury, taking their PhotoVoice Exhibit to various conferences, libraries and health care facilities. The project was even exhibited at the Massachusetts State House for Brain Injury Awareness Month and featured in the Boston Globe in March 2009!

When you feel ready to take on a project, I encourage you to consider doing a PhotoVoice Project; on your own, with another survivor friend or with your support group. I wish you an amazing journey and continued healing!

You may still be able to view the Framingham PhotoVoice Project on BIAMA.ORG (Support) or brainline.org (put PhotoVoice in the search box).

If you are interested in reading more about PhotoVoice as a research tool with brain injury survivors, please read Brain Injury Survivors: Narratives of Rehabilitation and Healing, by Laura S. Lorenz, PhD.

You might also like to include this journal article:
Lorenz, Laura S. (2010). Visual metaphors of living with brain injury: Exploring and communicating lived experience with an invisible injury, *Visual Studies*, 25(3), pp 210-223.

Doing Your Own PhotoVoice Project

Laura Lorenz, PhD and Barbara Webster

Adapted and reprinted with permission, Laura S. Lorenz

PhotoVoice is an activity that a brain injury survivor—or anyone—can do.

- ❏ On their own
- ❏ With a friend, family member, or rehabilitation service provider
- ❏ With a support group

Basically, PhotoVoice involves the following activities:

- ❏ Thinking of some questions you want to answer with your camera
- ❏ Taking pictures that answer your questions, from your perspective
- ❏ Reflecting on your pictures by yourself, or talking about your pictures with someone else
- ❏ Writing captions for some of your photos—you choose which ones!

PhotoVoice can include the following optional activities:

- ❏ Looking for themes in your photos and narratives and grouping them by theme
- ❏ Putting your photos and captions in a binder
- ❏ Sharing your binder with family, friends, and others—maybe a rehabilitation service provider!

The following pages will help you do your own PhotoVoice project:

- ❏ Getting Started
- ❏ PhotoVoice Tips!
- ❏ Photo-Taking Questions
- ❏ Photo-Taking Tips
- ❏ PhotoVoice Ethics: Safety and Respect!
- ❏ Photo Consent Form 1
- ❏ Photo Discussion Questions
- ❏ Building on Your PhotoVoice Project
- ❏ Exhibit Options
- ❏ Photo Consent Form 2

A Photovoice Path

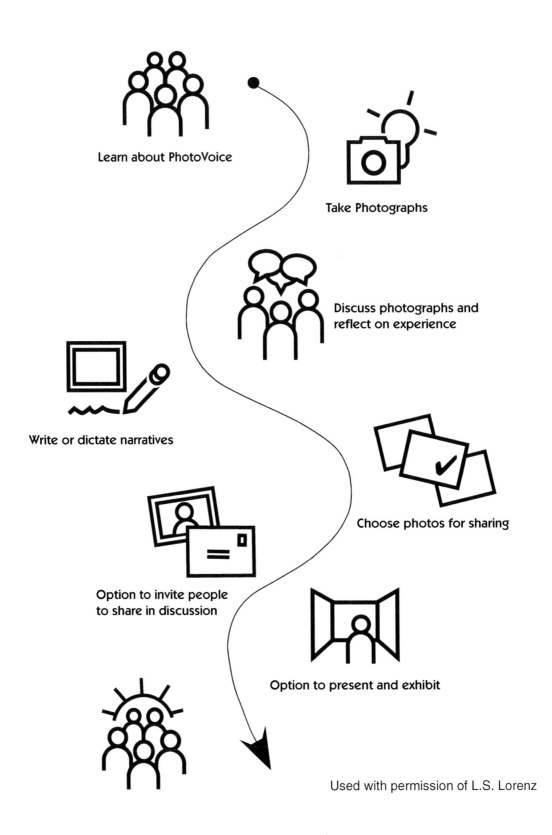

Learn about PhotoVoice

Take Photographs

Discuss photographs and reflect on experience

Write or dictate narratives

Choose photos for sharing

Option to invite people to share in discussion

Option to present and exhibit

Used with permission of L.S. Lorenz

Getting Started

Here is a list of steps to get you started doing your own PhotoVoice project:

1. Choose your camera. Any type of camera is fine. Most important is a camera that is easy for you to use.

2. Develop some questions you want to answer with your project. Investigate strengths as well as weaknesses—positives as well as negatives.

3. Reflect on how you might answer your questions using a photo. Write down ideas of pictures you would like to take. This is where using a notebook helps.

4. Take some photos. Write notes about why you took the picture if you like.

5. Look at your photos. Is there one that "speaks" to you? What do you see?

6. Write a caption for your chosen photo(s). Your caption can be short or long. Two or three sentences might be enough to tell your story.

7. Plan to take at least one more set of pictures. For most people, the first group of photos generates more ideas of photos. Learning how to illustrate your thoughts or feelings with photos and captions is an ongoing process!

PhotoVoice Tips

Keep these tips handy as you do your PhotoVoice project! Refer to them often.

No experience needed!

Owning a camera or having experience taking photographs is not necessary! For the Framingham Support Group project, we used inexpensive disposable cameras, but any camera will do.

Photo quality is not important.

PhotoVoice is not about the quality of your photographs. It is about taking pictures that mean something to you as a brain injury survivor.

Keep a notebook.

Write down ideas of photos in a notebook. Keep notes about why you took a picture.

Ask permission to take someone's photo.

Always ask permission before you take someone's picture! If they say no, explain briefly what you are doing and why you want to take their picture. Your explanation can simply be: "I'm working on a photography project for people with disabilities/ brain injuries, would you mind being in one of the photos?" If they still say no, take a picture of something or someone else instead!

File your photos.

Paste or glue each photo on a blank sheet of paper. Some people like to put two or three photos on one sheet. Remember to leave room for your caption, later. Place the sheets in a binder, for easy viewing and storing. OPTIONAL: Print two sets of photos, save the second set for future options.

Store your photo negatives or digital files where you can find them!

Keep your photo negatives (or a CD of your images) in a safe place, for making more prints later.

Write captions from your heart.

Write your captions as if you were talking to someone else about your photos. Speak from your heart. If writing is hard, dictate your captions to someone else to write down for you.

Photo-Taking Questions

These are the questions the Framingham Support Group used for their project. Feel free to use these questions, or develop new ones for yourself. Be sure to include questions that investigate strengths as well as weaknesses—positives as well as negatives.

- ❏ What is it like to live with brain injury?
- ❏ What in my life or community has helped me in my healing from brain injury?
- ❏ What in my life or community has slowed down my healing from brain injury?
- ❏ What do I want to tell other people about living with brain injury?
- ❏ How is my life different now than before? What is better? What is worse?
- ❏ What are my hopes for the future? And what might help me get there?

Photo-Taking Tips

Tips for taking good photographs

- ❏ Try different angles.
- ❏ Try different points of view.
- ❏ Keep the sun to your back, or to the side.
- ❏ Is your subject in the center of the photo?
- ❏ Does your subject fill the photo?

Tips for avoiding common mistakes

- ❏ Keep your finger away from the lens.
- ❏ Don't cover the flash.
- ❏ Stand about three to eight feet away from your subject.
- ❏ Wind the film forward before you take another picture.
- ❏ To prevent blurry pictures, hold your elbows close to your sides, and hold your breath when you press the shutter (button).

Please note: If you are using a film camera, you don't need to use the whole roll of film! Just take as many photos as you can or want to take. Even just 1 or 2 photos is okay. 5 or 6 is fine. 10 or 12 is a good number to start with if you can

PhotoVoice Ethics: Safety and Respect

With PhotoVoice, we are visual researchers as we take pictures of our lives with brain injury and talk about them with others.

As a visual researcher, you must keep certain guidelines in mind:

Stay safe!

Make sure you are "safe" when you take the picture. For example:

- ❏ Stand on a solid surface.
- ❏ Look before you step into or cross a street.
- ❏ Be aware of things around you, like traffic.

Ask permission.

Always ask permission before taking someone's photo for this project. Ask them to sign a photo consent form.

If someone can be recognized in a photo, ask permission before showing their picture outside your group.

Be respectful.

If someone doesn't want their photo taken, respect their feelings.

Be prepared.

Be ready to explain about the project to family, friends, or strangers, if they ask what you are doing.

A simple explanation is: "I am part of a PhotoVoice project investigating what it is like to live with brain injury. We are taking photographs of our lives and talking about them with other people in our group. Thank you for letting me take your picture."

When permission is not necessary.

In a public place like a park, you can take someone's photo without permission, especially if they are far away and can't be recognized in the picture.

Respect the lives and safety of others.

When you take photos for your project, think of people's safety first, and be respectful of their lives. For example:

- ❏ If your friend is diabetic and the doctor told him not to eat sweets, avoid taking a picture of him eating cake!
- ❏ If your friend doesn't have a driver's license, avoid taking a picture of her driving a car down the street!

Photo Discussion Questions

Here are some suggestions of questions to get you started talking about your photo with others—or for reflecting on your own:

❏ What does this photo show?

❏ What do you want to say about it?

❏ How does this help or slow down your healing from brain injury?

❏ What can we do to support healing from brain injury?

Building on Your Project

Many people have found that doing PhotoVoice helps to build their self-confidence and inspires them to take action to achieve another goal.
Is there another project you have been wanting to do?

❏ Pursue a hobby?

❏ Take a class?

❏ Start a garden?

❏ Start volunteering?

❏ Look into part-time work opportunities?

Think about how you might use your PhotoVoice project to take action on your goal. Building awareness about brain injury can become a goal. Your photos and captions might be the missing link to help people without brain injury to understand what it is like for you to live with a brain injury. Other brain injury survivors often feel validated in seeing your photos and captions, and having an opportunity to tell you their story in turn. One way to build on your project is to share your photos and captions with others.

Exhibit Options

An exhibit—for family, friends, or others—can be useful for telling your story. Be sure to include information about your project: what you did and why. Consider grouping your photos for display in categories of common themes.

Exhibit options can include:

❏ Mount your photos and captions on a flip chart or a poster board.

❏ Paste prints of your photos on colored paper along with their narratives. Laminate the pages for mounting on a wall or in a case, or for sharing.

❏ Frame some photos and hang them on a wall, with the captions in the frame or nearby.

❏ Prepare a slide show of your photos and captions in PowerPoint (or another software program). Record yourself reading your captions or talking about your pictures, if you like.

❏ Create a web site of your photos and captions

<u>Locations that might be interested in knowing about your exhibit could include:</u>

- ❏ Your local public library
- ❏ A coffee shop or book store that hosts exhibits of local artists
- ❏ Your state Brain Injury Association affiliate
- ❏ A medical center, rehabilitation center, or doctor's office
- ❏ A local senior or community center
- ❏ A local school

<u>Ask permission before including photos in an exhibit!</u>

If you are organizing an exhibit, obtain permission from each photographer before putting their photos in the exhibit. If the photographer does not want their photo(s) included, respect their wishes.

Photo Consent Form 1

I am part of a PhotoVoice project investigating what it is like to live with brain injury. We are taking photographs of our lives and talking about them with other people in our group.

Please sign this form if you agree to let me take your photograph for this project.

If you would like a copy of this photo, please write down your address.

I agree to have my photo taken for this PhotoVoice project:

_____

Name

_____

Signature

_____

Date

_____

Name of photographer

Photo Consent Form 2

I've been taking photographs of my experience living with brain injury.
With this form I give - or refuse - permission for my photos and captions to be used in a public display.

❏ Yes, I am willing to have my photographs and captions used in public displays about living with brain injury.

❏ No, I do not want my photographs and captions used in public displays about living with brain injury.

❏ I also need to give—or refuse—permission for my name to be listed as the photographer.

❏ I want my FULL NAME listed as the photographer.

❏ I want only my FIRST NAME listed as the photographer.

❏ I want only my INITIALS listed as the photographer.

❏ I DO NOT want my name listed at all.

Please list any concerns or comments:

_____

_____

_____

_____

_____

Name

_____

Signature

_____

Date

Tool Chest

Tool Templates

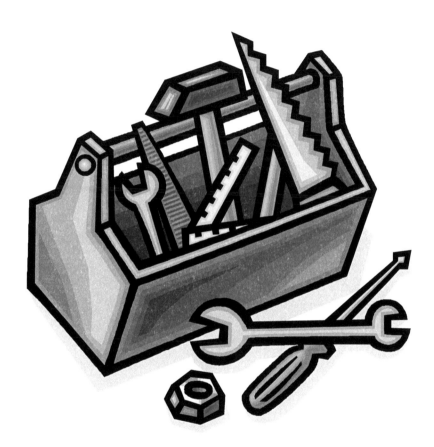

Inventory of Tool Templates

Please make copies of any tools you find helpful.

What Brain Injury Survivors Want You to Know

I need a lot more rest than I used to. I'm not being lazy. I get physical fatigue as well as a "brain fatigue". It is very difficult and tiring for my brain to think, process and organize. Fatigue makes it even harder to think.

My stamina fluctuates, even though I may look good or "all better" on the outside. Cognition is a fragile function for a brain injury survivor. Some days are better than others. Pushing too hard usually leads to setbacks, sometimes to illness.

Brain injury rehabilitation takes a very long time; it is usually measured in years. It continues long after formal rehabilitation has ended. Please resist expecting me to be who I was, even though I look better.

I am not being difficult if I resist social situations. Crowds, confusion and loud sounds quickly overload my brain, it doesn't filter sounds as well as it used to. Limiting my exposure is a coping strategy, not a behavioral problem.

If there is more than one person talking, I may seem uninterested in the conversation. That is because I have trouble following all the different "lines" of discussion. It is exhausting to keep trying to piece it all together. I'm not dumb or rude; my brain is getting overloaded!

If we are talking and I tell you that I need to stop, I need to stop NOW! And it is not because I'm avoiding the subject, it's just that I need time to process our discussion and "take a break" from all the thinking. Later I will be able to rejoin the conversation and really be present for the subject and for you.

Try to notice the circumstances if a behavior problem arises. "Behavior problems" are often an indication of my inability to cope with a specific situation and not a mental health issue. I may be frustrated, in pain, overtired or there may be too much confusion or noise for my brain to filter.

Patience is the best gift you can give me. It allows me to work deliberately and at my own pace, allowing me to rebuild pathways in my brain. Rushing and multi-tasking inhibit cognition.

Please listen to me with patience. Try not to interrupt. Allow me to find my words and follow my thoughts. It will help me rebuild my language skills.

Please have patience with my memory. Know that not remembering does not mean that I don't care.

Please don't be condescending or talk to me like I am a child. I'm not stupid, my brain is injured and it doesn't work as well as it used to. Try to think of me as if my brain were in a cast.

If I seem "rigid", needing to do tasks the same way all the time; it is because I am retraining my brain. It's like learning main roads before you can learn the shortcuts. Repeating tasks in the same sequence is a rehabilitation strategy.

If I seem "stuck", my brain may be stuck in the processing of information. Coaching me, suggesting other options or asking what you can do to help may help me figure it out. Taking over and doing it for me will not be constructive and it will make me feel inadequate. (It may also be an indication that I need to take a break.)

You may not be able to help me do something if helping requires me to frequently interrupt what I am doing to give you directives. I work best on my own, one step at a time and at my own pace.

If I repeat actions, like checking to see if the doors are locked or the stove is turned off, it may seem like I have OCD, obsessive-compulsive disorder but I may not. It may be that I am having trouble registering what I am doing in my brain. Repetitions enhance memory. (It can also be a cue that I need to stop and rest.)

If I seem sensitive, it could be emotional lability as a result of the injury or it may be a reflection of the extraordinary effort it takes to do things now. Tasks that used to feel "automatic" and take minimal effort, now take much longer, require the implementation of numerous strategies and are huge accomplishments for me.

We need cheerleaders now, as we start over, just like children do when they are growing up. Please help me and encourage all efforts. Please don't be negative or critical. I am doing the best I can.

Don't confuse Hope for Denial. We are learning more and more about the amazing brain and there are remarkable stories about healing in the news every day. No one can know for certain what our potential is. We need Hope to be able to employ the many, many coping mechanisms, accommodations and strategies needed to navigate our new lives. Everything single thing in our lives is extraordinarily difficult for us now. It would be easy to give up without Hope.

Created with the assistance of the
'Amazing' Brain Injury Survivor Support Group of Framingham, MA